Improving Care to Prevent Suicide Among People with Serious Mental Illness

PROCEEDINGS OF A WORKSHOP

Steve Olson, *Rapporteur*

Board on Health Care Services

Health and Medicine Division

Board on Children, Youth, and Families

Division of Behavioral and Social Sciences and Education

The National Academies of
SCIENCES · ENGINEERING · MEDICINE

THE NATIONAL ACADEMIES PRESS
Washington, DC
www.nap.edu

THE NATIONAL ACADEMIES PRESS   500 Fifth Street, NW   Washington, DC 20001

This activity was supported by the Substance Abuse and Mental Health Services Administration (Task Order 283-12-6101). Any opinions, findings, conclusions, or recommendations expressed in this publication do not necessarily reflect the views of any organization or agency that provided support for the project.

International Standard Book Number-13: 978-0-309-48694-1
International Standard Book Number-10: 0-309-48694-7
Digital Object Identifier: https://doi.org/10.17226/25318

Additional copies of this publication are available from the National Academies Press, 500 Fifth Street, NW, Keck 360, Washington, DC 20001; (800) 624-6242 or (202) 334-3313; http://www.nap.edu.

Copyright 2019 by the National Academy of Sciences. All rights reserved.

Printed in the United States of America

Suggested citation: National Academies of Sciences, Engineering, and Medicine. 2019. *Improving care to prevent suicide among people with serious mental illness: Proceedings of a workshop.* Washington, DC: The National Academies Press. doi: https://doi.org/10.17226/25318.

The National Academies of
SCIENCES • ENGINEERING • MEDICINE

The **National Academy of Sciences** was established in 1863 by an Act of Congress, signed by President Lincoln, as a private, nongovernmental institution to advise the nation on issues related to science and technology. Members are elected by their peers for outstanding contributions to research. Dr. Marcia McNutt is president.

The **National Academy of Engineering** was established in 1964 under the charter of the National Academy of Sciences to bring the practices of engineering to advising the nation. Members are elected by their peers for extraordinary contributions to engineering. Dr. C. D. Mote, Jr., is president.

The **National Academy of Medicine** (formerly the Institute of Medicine) was established in 1970 under the charter of the National Academy of Sciences to advise the nation on medical and health issues. Members are elected by their peers for distinguished contributions to medicine and health. Dr. Victor J. Dzau is president.

The three Academies work together as the **National Academies of Sciences, Engineering, and Medicine** to provide independent, objective analysis and advice to the nation and conduct other activities to solve complex problems and inform public policy decisions. The National Academies also encourage education and research, recognize outstanding contributions to knowledge, and increase public understanding in matters of science, engineering, and medicine.

Learn more about the National Academies of Sciences, Engineering, and Medicine at **www.nationalacademies.org**.

The National Academies of
SCIENCES • ENGINEERING • MEDICINE

Consensus Study Reports published by the National Academies of Sciences, Engineering, and Medicine document the evidence-based consensus on the study's statement of task by an authoring committee of experts. Reports typically include findings, conclusions, and recommendations based on information gathered by the committee and the committee's deliberations. Each report has been subjected to a rigorous and independent peer-review process and it represents the position of the National Academies on the statement of task.

Proceedings published by the National Academies of Sciences, Engineering, and Medicine chronicle the presentations and discussions at a workshop, symposium, or other event convened by the National Academies. The statements and opinions contained in proceedings are those of the participants and are not endorsed by other participants, the planning committee, or the National Academies.

For information about other products and activities of the National Academies, please visit www.nationalacademies.org/about/whatwedo.

PLANNING COMMITTEE ON IMPROVING CARE TO PREVENT SUICIDE AMONG PEOPLE WITH SERIOUS MENTAL ILLNESS[1]

M. DAVID RUDD (*Chair*), President, University of Memphis
TERESA BROCKIE, Assistant Professor, Community Public Health Nursing, School of Nursing, Johns Hopkins University
M. JUSTIN COFFEY, Vice President and Chief Information Officer, The Menninger Clinic
CHELSEY GODDARD, Vice President, Education Development Center, Inc.
AIMEE C. JOHNSON, Program Specialist, Public Private Partnerships, Office of Mental Health and Suicide Prevention, Veterans Health Administration, Portland Veterans Affairs Medical Center
NADINE KASLOW, Professor, Department of Psychiatry and Behavioral Science, School of Medicine, Emory University
ANDREY OSTROVSKY, Chief Executive Officer, Concerted Care Group

Project Staff

MARC MEISNERE, Associate Program Officer
JOSEPH GOODMAN, Senior Program Assistant
WENDY KEENAN, Program Officer (*until July 2018*)
NATALIE PEROU LUBIN, Senior Program Assistant (*from September 2018*)
SHARYL J. NASS, Director, Board on Health Care Services
NATACHA BLAIN, Director, Board on Children, Youth, and Families

Consultant

BRIDGET B. KELLY, Principal Consultant, Burke Kelly, Inc.

---

[1] The National Academies of Sciences, Engineering, and Medicine's planning committees are solely responsible for organizing the workshop, identifying topics, and choosing speakers. The responsibility for the published Proceedings of a Workshop rests with the workshop rapporteur and the institution.

Reviewers

This Proceedings of a Workshop was reviewed in draft form by individuals chosen for their diverse perspectives and technical expertise. The purpose of this independent review is to provide candid and critical comments that will assist the National Academies of Sciences, Engineering, and Medicine in making each published proceedings as sound as possible and to ensure that it meets the institutional standards for quality, objectivity, evidence, and responsiveness to the charge. The review comments and draft manuscript remain confidential to protect the integrity of the process.

We thank the following individuals for their review of this proceedings:

GRETCHEN HAAS, University of Pittsburgh
MIKE HOGAN, Hogan Health Solutions
KEITH WOOD, Emory University School of Medicine

Although the reviewers listed above provided many constructive comments and suggestions, they were not asked to endorse the content of the proceedings nor did they see the final draft before its release. The review of this proceedings was overseen by **PATRICK DELEON,** Uniformed Services University of the Health Sciences. He was responsible for making certain that an independent examination of this proceedings was carried out in accordance with standards of the National Academies and that all review comments were carefully considered. Responsibility for the final content rests entirely with the rapporteur and the National Academies.

Contents

1	INTRODUCTION AND OVERVIEW	1
2	PATTERNS OF RISK AND THE PREVENTION LANDSCAPE	9
3	SUICIDE PREVENTION IN HEALTH CARE SYSTEMS	29
4	MILITARY SERVICE MEMBERS AND VETERANS	45
5	NATIVE AMERICANS AND ALASKA NATIVES	57
6	CONNECTING PREVENTION ALONG THE CONTINUUM OF CARE	71
7	PERSPECTIVES ON THE FUTURE ALONG THE CONTINUUM	81
8	IDEAS FROM THE BREAKOUT SESSIONS	91
9	REFLECTIONS ON THE WORKSHOP	97

APPENDIXES

A	WORKSHOP AGENDA	103
B	BIOGRAPHICAL SKETCHES	107

1

Introduction and Overview[1]

On October 5, 2002, Taryn Hiatt, a founding member of the Utah chapter and area director for Utah and Nevada of the American Foundation for Suicide Prevention, lost her father to suicide. He had lived with serious mental illness that went untreated for most of his life. Her family knew that he was ill. Over the course of his life, he had more than 22 surgeries to treat his esophagus from the effects of acid reflux. In the weeks before his suicide, he was taking 30 Ambien per day in addition to a variety of other medications. "His depression was always treated with medication," Hiatt said, some of which were probably needed and some of which were probably not needed. But, Hiatt added, he never received any behavioral treatments so that he would better understand what he was grappling with, and neither did his family.

Hiatt's father was ashamed "for having an illness that he thought was somehow his fault," she said. After his death, her family was ashamed, too. They wondered what to tell people. They talked about whether they should say he had died from a heart attack. "I remember saying no," said Hiatt. "I wanted to share the word. We're done doing this. We're done being quiet."

On September 11–12, 2018, the National Academies of Sciences, Engineering, and Medicine (the National Academies) held a workshop in

---

[1] The planning committee's role was limited to planning the workshop, and the Proceedings of a Workshop was prepared by the workshop rapporteur as a factual summary of what occurred at the workshop. Statements, recommendations, and opinions expressed are those of individual presenters and participants, and are not necessarily endorsed or verified by the National Academies of Sciences, Engineering, and Medicine, and they should not be construed as reflecting any group consensus.

Washington, DC, to discuss an issue that could have saved Hiatt's father and the lives of thousands of other people every year in the United States: preventing suicide among people with serious mental illness. Suicide prevention initiatives are part of much broader systems, said David Rudd, president of the University of Memphis and member of the workshop planning committee. Such initiatives are connected to activities like the diagnosis of mental illness, the recognition of clinical risk, improving access to care, and coordinating with a broad range of outside agencies and entities around both prevention and public health efforts. Yet, suicide is also an intensely personal issue that continues to be surrounded by stigma, Rudd pointed out. "Sometimes it is hard to remember that behind every number is a person, is a family, is a network, and that many people and many lives are touched in each and every one of these instances." It is a national problem, he said, yet it remains hard to have these conversations. "I can think of case after case after case where we have a difficult time saying *suicide*."

The workshop was designed to illustrate and discuss what is known, what is currently being done, and what needs to be done to identify and reduce suicide risk among people with serious mental illness. Box 1-1 provides the workshop Statement of Task. Appendix A contains the workshop agenda and Appendix B provides biographical sketches of

---

BOX 1-1
Workshop Statement of Task

The workshop presentations and moderated discussions will examine opportunities to prevent suicide among people with serious mental illness (SMI), including, at minimum, bipolar disorder, major depression, schizophrenia, and borderline personality disorder, as well as mood, anxiety, or other disorders that result in significant functional impairment.

The workshop will:

- Highlight the patterns of mortality by suicide among people with SMI,
- Consider the implications of the relationship between SMI and suicide, and
- Examine interventions that can reduce the high risk of suicide in this population.

The workshop will also consider ways to:

- Improve and implement early interventions,
- Improve access to care among vulnerable populations with SMI, and
- Effectively target interventions to specific populations with unique needs.

the workshop speakers, panelists, facilitators, planning committee members, staff, and consultants. A video archive of the workshop can be accessed on the Health and Medicine Division of the National Academies' project page.[2]

THE NEED FOR INFORMATION AND COMMUNICATION

Individuals and families need the same education to prevent suicide that they would receive for other health issues, Hiatt said in her presentation during the opening session of the workshop. If her father had been living with cancer, diabetes, dementia, or Alzheimer's, Hiatt noted, his family would have received the information they needed to support him and encourage him to get the help that he needed. But they did not receive the information they needed. Today, others reach out to Hiatt for help, and she refers them to the resources that are available. "But we need more," she said, adding:

> I love the movement that's taking place in our nation where we're finally addressing suicide as a health issue. But, again, if we're going to treat it as the health issue it is, we need to do that on all aspects. There's no shame in getting help for it. There's no shame in admitting that that's what I'm thinking.

Suicidal behavior is an attempt to cope, as is all behavior, she said. A person in that moment of intense pain and crisis has a belief system that is altered. The workshop began on September 11, and she drew an analogy to the event that occurred 17 years earlier on that date. As the Twin Towers in New York City began to burn, people at the tops of the towers began to jump.

By definition, they took their own life. They died of suicide. Yet, none of us sat on our couch and said, "Oh my gosh, you coward, how selfish of you. How could you do that to your friends and family?" Did they jump because they wanted to die? No. They jumped because they were desperate to escape pain and anguish. They jumped because their thinking was anything but rational in that moment and their crisis point had been reached.

People who are thinking of suicide need the same level of compassion, Hiatt said. They have reached a point where they feel they cannot live, whether because of their mental illness, their life experiences, or their trauma. Hiatt made her own suicide attempts as a teenager, she said. "I understand what it's like to live in that dark night of the soul." When she

---

[2] See http://nationalacademies.org/hmd/Activities/MentalHealth/SuicidePreventionMentalIllness/2018-Sep-11/Videos/Opening-Videos/1-Welcome-Video.aspx (accessed November 27, 2018).

tried to end her life as a teenager, she did not want to die, but she did not know how to live with what was happening to her. Yet, she survived and has gone on to live a full and meaningful life. "There's hope in that. There's hope for recovery, and that's the message we need to continue to get out there. Suicide can be prevented."

Everyone needs to know the warning signs for suicide the same way they know the signs for heart attacks and strokes, she observed. Everyone needs to be capable and willing to administer the care that people need in their moments of crisis. Her father is someone who would have benefited from the sharing of electronic health records, Hiatt said, so that the emergency room doctor he saw on the day of his suicide would have seen that he had attempted suicide before and that he was getting medications from multiple doctors. It would have been an opportunity, she added, for a physician to talk with him about his pain and not simply prescribe the medications that he used to end his own life. Hiatt now has her own suicide safety plan. When she needs help, she gets in to see a therapist.

A few weeks before the workshop, the Church of Jesus Christ of Latter-day Saints in Utah, where Hiatt lives, said that it will no longer consider suicide a sin. Crying in her car when she heard the news, Hiatt was immensely grateful for the progress of recent decades that made such a decision possible. But she also recalled that society continues to put a great burden on suicidal individuals. "We're talking about a person who's desperate to escape unbearable pain." Telling them not to take their own lives, she observed, is like telling someone with cancer to choose to live without giving them the tools, treatment, and care they need to do that.

"I decided 16 years ago I wasn't going to rest until we stopped suicide," Hiatt said. "I want this to no longer be the health issue of our time. We do that by these conversations. We do that by taking note. We do that by creating awareness. We're aware suicide is a problem. We need to take action."

SUPPORT FOR THE WORKSHOP

Richard McKeon, chief of the Suicide Prevention Branch in the Center for Mental Health Services, Substance Abuse and Mental Health Services Administration (SAMHSA), briefly spoke about why SAMHSA supported the workshop. Suicide rates have increased significantly in the United States in recent years, he observed. A recent report from the Centers for Disease Control and Prevention (CDC) showed that suicide had increased in 49 of 50 states between 1999 and 2016, and in half the states examined the increase was greater than 30 percent (Stone et al., 2018). "There is clearly a need for us to do more and better," said McKeon, "to increase the effectiveness of our suicide prevention efforts and to try to save as many lives as possible."

Rates of suicide are significantly elevated among those with serious mental illness and serious emotional disturbance, McKeon observed. This has practical implications for SAMHSA, since its mental health programs are by statute required to focus on adults with serious mental illness or youth with serious emotional disturbance. Currently, SAMHSA has an array of suicide prevention initiatives. These include support for the Zero Suicide approach described in Chapter 2. SAMHSA recently made 14 suicide prevention grants to states, health care systems, and tribes. It also has a significant youth suicide prevention initiative, the Garrett Lee Smith grants, that have gone over the past 12 years to each of the 50 states.

SAMHSA is interested in identifying those who are at risk for suicide who may also experience serious emotional disturbance, how best to intervene with them once they are engaged in the health care system, and what are the best approaches to use. These "are vitally important issues for SAMHSA," said McKeon, and he welcomed the "advice, guidance, wisdom, and discussion that I'm sure all of you will provide."

OVERVIEW OF THE WORKSHOP

The workshop consisted of six plenary panel presentations, a breakout session on the second day, and opportunities to report back from the breakout sessions and comment on the major themes and messages that emerged from the workshop.

In the first panel presentation, which is summarized in Chapter 2, Holly Wilcox, associate professor in the Johns Hopkins Bloomberg School of Public Health's Department of Mental Health and the Johns Hopkins University School of Medicine's Department of Psychiatry, and Christine Moutier, chief medical officer of the American Foundation for Suicide Prevention, provided broad overviews of the prevalence of suicide, changes in prevalence over time, and the links between suicide and serious mental illness. Critical windows exist for suicide risk, such as the week after discharge from a psychiatric admission or emergency department presentation for suicidal ideation or attempt, the first weeks after starting an antidepressant, and during significant life transitions. Both universal and targeted interventions have proven effective in improving suicide rates, but they require continued support and attention to the quality of implementation, the presenters observed.

During the second panel (summarized in Chapter 3), C. Edward Coffey, professor of psychiatry and behavioral sciences and of neurology in the Baylor College of Medicine, traced the origins of the Zero Suicide movement back to the 2001 Institute of Medicine (IOM) report *Crossing the Quality Chasm: A New Health System for the 21st Century*. Initially successful at the Henry Ford Health System, this approach, which uses a care protocol for suicide risk and quality improvement principles, has since been adopted in other locations around the world, as pointed out by David Covington, chief executive officer and president of Recovery Innovations, Inc. It is an especially effective way, noted Mike Hogan of Hogan Health Solutions, to ensure that people with suicidality do not make their way through successive gaps in care and to integrate care for those with both serious mental illness and suicidality.

The third and fourth panels of the workshop looked at two groups at high risk for suicide: military service members and veterans, and American Indians and Alaska Natives. In the third panel (summarized in Chapter 4), both Mike Colston, captain in the U.S. Navy Medical Corps and director of Mental Health Programs in the Health Services and Policy Oversight Office of the Department of Defense, and Keita Franklin, national director of suicide prevention for the Office of Mental Health and Suicide Prevention in the Department of Veterans Affairs (VA), pointed out that the suicide rate among active duty service members has increased in recent decades. Colson described the range of effective interventions that are now available that can save lives. Franklin discussed the universal, selective, and indicated prevention components of a comprehensive public health campaign to prevent suicide among veterans. She also advocated for a "whole of government" and "whole of industry" approach that could coordinate and intensify suicide prevention work with this population, including those veterans who are not enrolled in care with the Veterans Health Administration.

The next panel (summarized in Chapter 5) considered Native American and American Indian communities, many of which have especially high levels of unmet health needs. The panel highlighted examples of approaches for suicide prevention and mental health in both communities and health systems. All four presenters—James Allen, professor in the Department of Family Medicine and Biobehavioral Health at the University of Minnesota Medical School; Allison Barlow, director of the Johns Hopkins Center for American Indian Health; Laurelle Myhra, director of behavioral health at the Native American Community Clinic; and Jennifer Shaw, a senior researcher at Southcentral Foundation—made the point that effective suicide prevention is culturally tailored to the population it serves. Shaw, for example, observed that interventions need to be targeted at all levels of human experience, respect autonomy, and honor community, which requires that they be tailored to or developed from within local cultures and patterns of being, communication, and relationship. In addition, Myhra noted that meeting the mental health needs of Native communities requires workforce development, including the training of Native behavioral health providers, community health workers, and people who can provide peer support.

In the fifth panel (summarized in Chapter 6), Nikole Jones, a suicide prevention coordinator with the VA Maryland Health Care System; Alfreda

Patterson, a substance use counselor and housing coordinator with Concerted Care Group in Baltimore; T. J. Wocasek, a clinical supervisor for the Southcentral Foundation in Anchorage, Alaska; and Keith Wood, clinical director of an intensive outpatient service with Emory University School of Medicine, described the approaches they and their organizations take toward individuals with suicidality, including those with serious mental illness. Several of the presenters had their own personal experiences with suicide, which have served as a guide and inspiration for them in developing relationships with their clients.

The final panel (summarized in Chapter 7) offered perspectives ranging from the direct patient experience of systems of care and outreach to the design of behavioral health systems at the state and city levels. Marcus Lilly, an outreach worker for Concerted Care Group, observed that partnerships between health care providers, mental health services providers, and community-based self-help groups could increase the availability of suicide prevention services and provide for long-term comprehensive treatment. Julie Goldstein Grumet, director of health and behavioral health initiatives at the Suicide Prevention Resource Center and director of the Zero Suicide Institute at Education Development Center, pointed out that investments both upstream and downstream from suicide prevention could link public health and mental health. Arthur Evans, chief executive officer of the American Psychological Association and previously the commissioner in Philadelphia for the Department of Behavioral Health and Intellectual Disability Services, called for approaches that address the challenge at the levels of providers, systems, and the community. He also made the point that the implementation of evidence-based treatment, including provider training in suicide prevention for people with serious mental illness, will require substantial investments of resources.

On the second day of the workshop, participants broke into two sessions to discuss major issues that arose over the course of the first day's discussions. Participants in one session discussed the financing and other policy issues associated with integrating suicide prevention into care for people with serious mental illness. Participants in the other session discussed issues associated with a focus on what providers need, which also encompassed political leadership. Chapter 8 summarizes the reports from those breakout sessions and the discussion that followed in the subsequent plenary session.

The final session of the workshop (summarized in Chapter 9) provided an opportunity for workshop participants to identify what they considered to be important messages they were taking away from the workshop.

In a follow-up to the workshop, a Twitter chat was hosted on October 4, 2018, by the National Academies' Health and Medicine Division (@NASEM_Health). This was a moderated public discussion in real time tied to the hashtag #SuicidePreventionChat. It continued the conversation about the intersection between suicide prevention and serious mental illness. The following questions were posed to participants in the chat:

- How does what is known about how to prevent suicide need to be adapted for people with serious mental illness?
- What can be done to better equip providers in behavioral health and mental health care for suicide prevention?
- How can more comprehensive disposition planning and follow-up after acute crises help stop suicide for those with serious mental illness?
- How can health systems improve tracking of suicide-related outcomes to inform better care for those with serious mental illness?
- What is your key message about improving suicide prevention for those with serious mental illness?

A link to the chat can be found on the website of the National Academies' Health and Medicine Division.[3]

REFERENCE

Stone, D. M., T. R. Simon, K. A. Fowler, S. R. Kegler, K. Yuan, K. M. Holland, A. Z. Ivey-Stephenson, and A. E. Crosby. 2018. Vital signs: Trends in state suicide rates—United States, 1999-2016 and circumstances contributing to suicide—27 States, 2015. *Morbidity and Mortality Weekly Report* 67(22):617-624.

---

[3] See http://nationalacademies.org/hmd/Activities/MentalHealth/SuicidePreventionMentalIllness/2018-Sep-11/twitter-chat-suicide-prevention.aspx (accessed November 27, 2018).

2

Patterns of Risk and the Prevention Landscape

Points Made by the Presenters

- Rates of suicide in the United States have ranged from 10 to 13 per 100,000 people for decades with a recent steady increase. (Wilcox)
- Several psychiatric conditions have been linked with suicide. (Wilcox)
- Psychological autopsy studies show that around 90 percent of those who die by suicide would meet criteria for at least one mental disorder. (Wilcox)
- Critical windows exist for suicide risk, such as the week after discharge from a psychiatric admission or emergency department presentation for suicidal ideation or attempt, the first weeks after starting an antidepressant, and during significant life transitions. (Moutier)
- Public health and health care system interventions have shown reductions in suicide rates in the United States and other countries, though they require continued support and attention to the quality of implementation. (Wilcox)
- Innovations in clinical treatments, including psychotherapies and medication, have increased the potential effectiveness of suicide prevention, including among those with serious mental illness. (Moutier)

- The most promising approach is to maximize optimal management of primary psychiatric conditions and to specifically consider suicide. (Moutier).
- The suicide prevention movement has been gaining momentum as organizations, advocates, and others have increasingly spoken out and as organizations have collaborated on effective strategies. (Moutier)

NOTE: These points were made by the individual workshop presenters identified above. They are not intended to reflect a consensus among workshop participants.

Suicide is the 10th leading cause of death in the United States (see Figure 2-1), and among young people ages 10 through 34 it is the second leading cause, observed Holly Wilcox, associate professor in the Johns Hopkins Bloomberg School of Public Health's Department of Mental Health and the Johns Hopkins University School of Medicine's Department of Psychiatry, in her overview of patterns of risk and the prevention landscape at the workshop. Beginning in adolescence, which is also an important developmental stage for the onset of mental illness, suicide becomes more common in males than in females (see Figure 2-2). In contrast, women typically report more suicide attempts than men. Men are more likely to use highly lethal means in a suicide attempt such as firearms. The economic impact of suicidal behaviors has been estimated to exceed $90 billion annually in the United States, mostly due to lost productivity (Shepard et al., 2016).

Firearms account for the majority of suicides in the United States (see Figure 2-3), and 60 percent of firearm deaths are by suicide. A promising new development, said Wilcox, is that 13 states have current legislation planned or in place for extreme risk protection orders, which give family members, first responders, and, in some instances, health care professionals the opportunity to petition to restrict purchase or possession of firearms by those who are deemed to be dangerous to self or others.

Case and Deaton (2017) found that the cohort of Americans who were born around 1950 and entered the workforce around 1970 have had particularly high suicide rates, which points to the toll that economic conditions may have on suicide risk, said Wilcox. This increase has been especially notable for men and women with a high school degree or less, though the rates have also increased, although to a lesser extent, for people with a 4-year college degree or more. To illustrate this point, Wilcox presented Figure 2-4.

According to data from the Centers for Disease Control and Prevention (CDC), the number of suicides in the year 2016 in the United States was approximately 45,000 (Stone et al., 2018). Stone et al. (2018) using

10 Leading Causes of Death by Age Group, United States – 2016

Rank	<1	1-4	5-9	10-14	15-24	25-34	35-44	45-54	55-64	65+	Total
1	Congenital Anomalies 4,816	Unintentional Injury 1,261	Unintentional Injury 787	Unintentional Injury 847	Unintentional Injury 13,895	Unintentional Injury 23,984	Unintentional Injury 20,975	Malignant Neoplasms 41,291	Malignant Neoplasms 116,364	Heart Disease 507,118	Heart Disease 635,260
2	Short Gestation 3,927	Congenital Anomalies 433	Malignant Neoplasms 449	Suicide 436	Suicide 5,723	Suicide 7,366	Malignant Neoplasms 10,903	Heart Disease 34,027	Heart Disease 78,610	Malignant Neoplasms 422,927	Malignant Neoplasms 598,038
3	SIDS 1,500	Malignant Neoplasms 377	Congenital Anomalies 203	Malignant Neoplasms 431	Homicide 5,172	Homicide 5,376	Heart Disease 10,477	Unintentional Injury 23,377	Unintentional Injury 21,860	Chronic Low. Respiratory Disease 131,002	Unintentional Injury 161,374
4	Maternal Pregnancy Comp. 1,402	Homicide 339	Homicide 139	Homicide 147	Malignant Neoplasms 1,431	Malignant Neoplasms 3,791	Suicide 7,030	Suicide 8,437	Chronic Low. Respiratory Disease 17,810	Cerebro-vascular 121,630	Chronic Low. Respiratory Disease 154,596
5	Unintentional Injury 1,219	Heart Disease 118	Heart Disease 77	Congenital Anomalies 146	Heart Disease 949	Heart Disease 3,445	Homicide 3,369	Liver Disease 8,364	Diabetes Mellitus 14,251	Alzheimer's Disease 114,883	Cerebro-vascular 142,142
6	Placenta Cord. Membranes 841	Influenza & Pneumonia 103	Chronic Low. Respiratory Disease 68	Heart Disease 111	Congenital Anomalies 388	Liver Disease 925	Liver Disease 2,851	Diabetes Mellitus 6,267	Liver Disease 13,448	Diabetes Mellitus 56,452	Alzheimer's Disease 116,103
7	Bacterial Sepsis 583	Septicemia 70	Influenza & Pneumonia 48	Chronic Low. Respiratory Disease 75	Diabetes Mellitus 211	Diabetes Mellitus 792	Diabetes Mellitus 2,049	Cerebro-vascular 5,353	Cerebro-vascular 12,310	Unintentional Injury 53,141	Diabetes Mellitus 80,058
8	Respiratory Distress 488	Perinatal Period 60	Septicemia 40	Cerebro-vascular 50	Chronic Low Respiratory Disease 206	Cerebro-vascular 575	Cerebro-vascular 1,851	Chronic Low. Respiratory Disease 4,307	Suicide 7,759	Influenza & Pneumonia 42,479	Influenza & Pneumonia 51,537
9	Circulatory System Disease 460	Cerebro-vascular 55	Cerebro-vascular 38	Influenza & Pneumonia 39	Influenza & Pneumonia 189	HIV 546	HIV 971	Septicemia 2,472	Septicemia 5,941	Nephritis 41,095	Nephritis 50,046
10	Neonatal Hemorrhage 398	Chronic Low Respiratory Disease 51	Benign Neoplasms 31	Septicemia 31	Complicated Pregnancy 184	Complicated Pregnancy 472	Septicemia 897	Homicide 2,152	Nephritis 5,650	Septicemia 30,405	Suicide 44,965

FIGURE 2-1 Suicide is the 10th leading cause of death in the United States and the second leading cause among people ages 10 through 34.
NOTE: HIV = human immunodeficiency virus; SIDS = sudden infant death syndrome.
SOURCES: Presented by Holly Wilcox on September 11, 2018, at the Workshop on Improving Care to Prevent Suicide Among People with Serious Mental Illness. From Centers for Disease Control and Prevention Web-based Injury Statistics Query and Reporting System data.

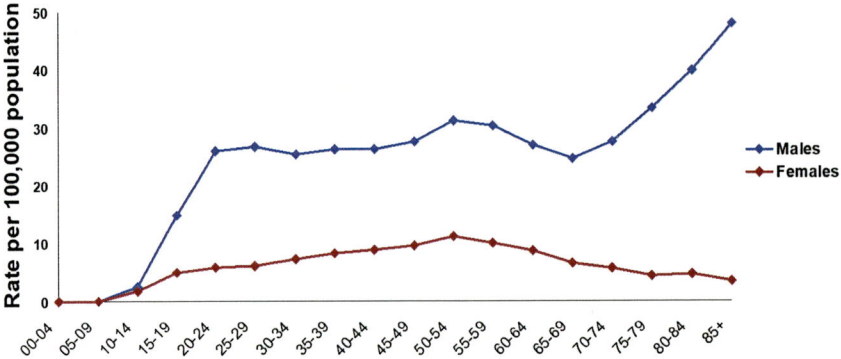

FIGURE 2-2 The suicide rate for men rises rapidly in adolescence and at older ages.
SOURCES: Presented by Holly Wilcox on September 11, 2018, at the Workshop on Improving Care to Prevent Suicide Among People with Serious Mental Illness. Data from National Vital Statistics System, National Center for Health Statistics, CDC.

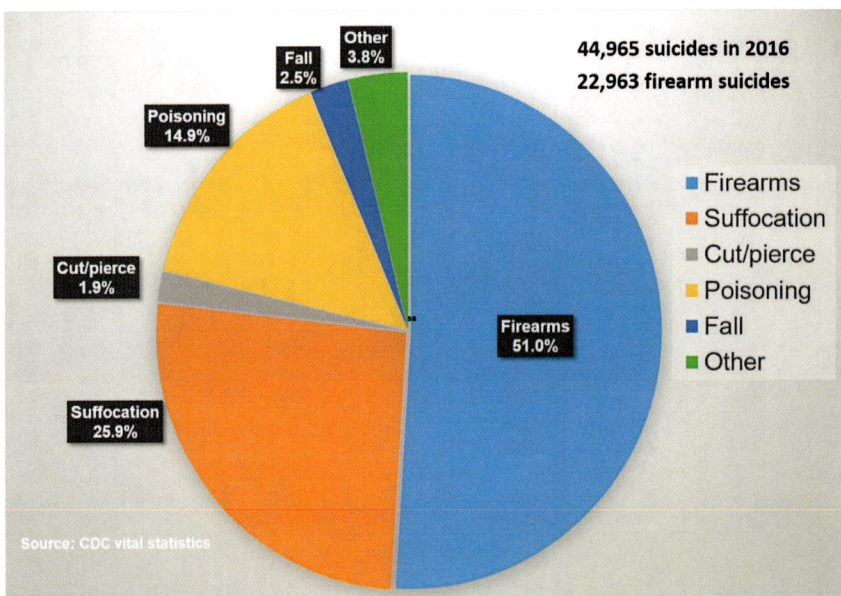

FIGURE 2-3 Firearms account for more than half of suicide deaths.
SOURCES: Presented by Holly Wilcox on September 11, 2018, at the Workshop on Improving Care to Prevent Suicide Among People with Serious Mental Illness. Data from National Vital Statistics System, National Center for Health Statistics, CDC.

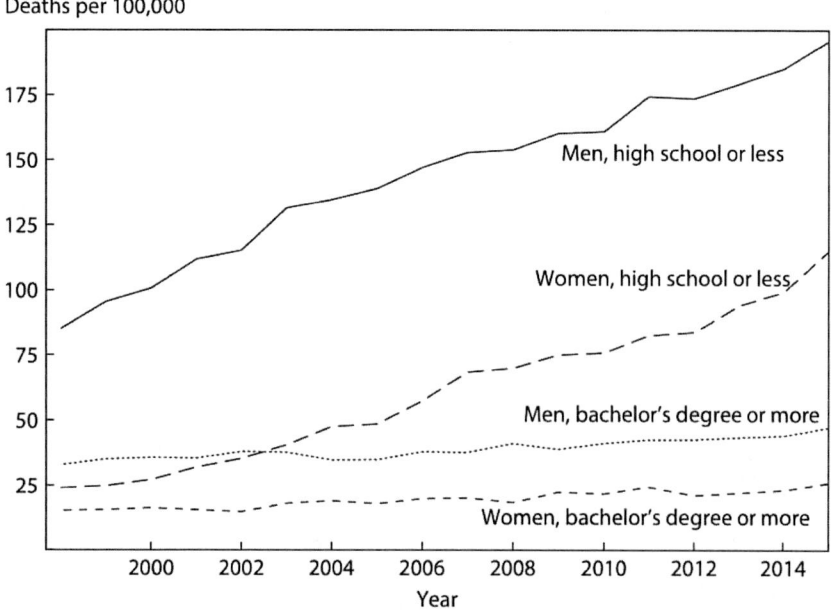

FIGURE 2-4 Middle-aged white mortality by suicide, drug overdose, or alcohol has risen rapidly over time.
SOURCES: Presented by Holly Wilcox on September 11, 2018, at the Workshop on Improving Care to Prevent Suicide Among People with Serious Mental Illness. From Case and Deaton (2017), used with permission.

the National Violent Death Reporting System to examine demographic and descriptive characteristics and contributing circumstances to suicide among people with and without known mental health conditions, found that suicide rates had increased by 30 percent or more since 1999 in more than half the 27 states examined. Stone et al. also found that, among those who died by suicide, 54 percent of people did not have a known mental health condition. This seemingly contradicts the conclusions from several studies based on psychological autopsy, Wilcox noted, which have found that more than 90 percent of people who die by suicide have at least one type of psychiatric disorder at the time of death, whether diagnosed or not (Cavanagh et al., 2003). Both are important pieces of information, and the actual number is likely somewhere in between, said Wilcox. The National Violent Death Reporting System does not actively assess for psychiatric status at the time of death, thus reflecting only what has otherwise been reported. When family members and others respond to psychological autopsies the information can indicate the presence of unreported psychiatric diagnoses, but in the context of losing a loved one to suicide family members may also overreport the extent of mental health concerns the individual had.

Studies that have examined the percentage of suicide attempts attributable to specific mental health disorders in nationally representative samples have noted that although many mental illnesses were associated with suicide attempts, elevated rates were mostly attributed to the presence of major depressive disorder, borderline personality disorder, nicotine dependence, and post-traumatic stress disorder (Bolton and Robinson, 2010). A whole population study from Sweden that studied risk for suicide after hospitalization for suicide attempts found that the risk and timing of suicide was particularly strong for people with unipolar and bipolar depression and schizophrenia, particularly among males (Tidemalm et al., 2008). This study underscored the need for more focused care during the first 2 years after a suicide attempt.

PUBLIC HEALTH AND SYSTEMS-LEVEL INITIATIVES

A public health initiative that was effective for a period of time in reducing suicides is the U.S. Air Force Suicide Prevention Program, said Wilcox. It is a comprehensive, system-level strategy with 11 components (Knox et al., 2010):

- Leadership involvement
- Professional military education
- Guidelines for commanders on use of mental health services
- Community preventive services
- Community education and training
- Investigative interview policy
- Trauma stress response team
- Integrated Delivery System (IDS) and Community Action Information Board (CAIB)
- Limited Privilege Suicide Prevention Program—Patients at risk for suicide are afforded increased confidentiality
- IDS Consultation Assessment Tool (originally the Behavioral Health Survey)
- Suicide Event Surveillance System

From a suicide rate in 1994 of 16.4 per 100,000 people, the rate dropped to 9.4 in 1998 after the suicide prevention program was implemented across the service. However, the rate went back up to 20.5 in 2015, despite the program's existence. This regression draws attention to the need for attention to the quality of implementation and continued support for interventions and monitoring, Wilcox said.

Another systems approach took place in the United Kingdom and included nine evidence-based components (While et al., 2012):

- Inpatient psychiatric unit safety
- Assertive outreach team
- 24/7 crisis team
- 7-day follow-up
- Written policy on nonadherence
- Dual diagnosis treatment
- Criminal justice sharing
- Debriefing and family contact after suicide
- Frontline clinical staff trained in management of suicide risk at least every 3 years

Mental health systems were encouraged to introduce as many of these components as possible. Those that implemented seven to nine components had significantly lower suicide rates than those implementing fewer components. Particularly effective approaches were 24-hour crisis teams that were able to intervene in crises, managing patients with dual diagnoses, and multidisciplinary reviews after suicides that shared information with families.

This work is especially relevant in the United States, as limited access to care is likely a contributing factor to the increasing U.S. suicide rate, Wilcox continued. The number of psychiatric beds in the United States has dropped in the past two decades even as the suicide rate has increased (Bastiampillai et al., 2016). This highlights the importance of high-quality community-based mental health services, said Wilcox.

Wilcox particularly emphasized the need to use data to inform suicide prevention. The combined effect of multiple risk and protective factors needs to be assessed in real time (Franklin et al., 2017). In addition, data linkage and predictive analytics with machine learning can identify those at risk and evaluate as well as identify the most effective policies and programs in reducing suicide, though privacy protection for individuals is a concern. Examples of projects using data to inform suicide prevention include approaches applied to U.S. veterans (McCarthy et al., 2015), the U.S. Army (Kessler et al., 2015; Nock et al., 2018), and health care patients (Tran et al., 2014; Simon et al., 2018).

Treatments targeting depression and anxiety in childhood and adolescence have been shown to reduce future risk for suicide ideation and attempts (March et al., 2006; Wolk et al., 2015). In addition, family and school-based universal prevention programs implemented as early as first grade reduce the incidence of suicidal ideation and attempt more than a decade later (Hawkins et al., 2005; Wilcox et al., 2008; Wasserman et al.,

2015; Connell et al., 2016). These interventions, Wilcox said, are highly practical, sustainable, and cost-effective and prevent multiple outcomes at a population level while producing cost savings for taxpayers and society.

Many policies and programs exist that simultaneously reduce or prevent addiction and multiple domains of violence, including suicide. Examples include evidence-based early childhood universal prevention programs (Hawkins et al., 2005; Wilcox et al., 2008; Connell et al., 2016); restricting firearm access, though vague definitions and enforcement can be challenging, Wilcox acknowledged (Kellerman et al., 1992; Miller and Hemenway, 2008; Miller et al., 2013; Anglemyer et al., 2014; Crifasi et al., 2015; Wintemute, 2015); maltreatment interventions such as early childhood home visitation programs (Hahn et al., 2003; Bilukha et al., 2005); and family-based policies such as divorce and child custody laws (Stevenson and Wolfers, 2006; Halla, 2013). A particular example Wilcox cited is the Good Behavior Game, which has demonstrated that it can reduce not only suicidal behaviors but other forms of violence and negative outcomes as well. Furthermore, the Good Behavior Game has been estimated to produce a return of more than $64 for every dollar invested in terms of long-term outcomes such as increases in high school graduation and prevention of the incidence of adverse mental health and behavioral outcomes.

Comprehensive system-wide programs can prevent suicide (Knox et al., 2003; McCarthy et al., 2009; While et al., 2012; Cwik et al., 2016), but they need to be embedded within systems to be sustained and they require attention to the quality of implementation, Wilcox said. Supportive contacts after being treated for a suicide attempt during the return to the community are also critical, with peer-to-peer approaches showing strong potential for being effective.

Wilcox also pointed out, in response to a question, that demonstrating the effect of specific suicide prevention programs can be difficult. Large studies are needed, since suicide is still a relatively infrequent outcome.

PERCEPTIONS AND AWARENESS OF SUICIDE PREVENTION

Public perceptions around mental health and suicide prevention have been undergoing dramatic changes, said Christine Moutier, chief medical officer of the American Foundation for Suicide Prevention, who also presented an overview of suicide prevention programs and policies during the workshop's first panel. First, the science informing mental health, psychology, psychiatry, neuroscience, and suicide has been growing rapidly in recent decades, and the results of that science are being disseminated and promoted much more actively. As just one example, the idea that mental health exists on a continuum, as for other aspects of health, is much more widely understood, though this idea still needs to be more widely disseminated, she said.

At the same time, the suicide prevention movement has gained momentum as organizations, advocates, and others who have who have been personally affected by suicide have spoken out. In addition, the field of suicide prevention is characterized by much more collaboration and consensus on effective strategies than has been the case in the past, which has helped shift public attitudes. According to a recent Harris poll sponsored by the American Foundation for Suicide Prevention and the National Action Alliance for Suicide Prevention, nearly 90 percent of people view physical and mental health as equally important, 93 percent of people would do something to help if someone close to them was thinking about suicide, and 96 percent of people think suicide is preventable. People also said that they would not be sure of what to do or say, Moutier added, so they need more knowledge.

Another shift Moutier identified as important is in the words people use to refer to suicide. In 2016 the Associated Press changed its stylebook. Its guidance is to avoid the phrase *commit suicide* and instead say *died by suicide* or *ended his or her life* and to say that someone attempted suicide instead of referring to a successful or failed suicide attempt. Another sign of a changed culture is rapid growth of the Out of the Darkness community, campus, and overnight walks, which began as a fledgling awareness and fundraising activity 15 years ago and have grown tremendously. "They started at a time when families and people were not sure that they could say the word *suicide* out loud in public," said Moutier. "Now hundreds of thousands of people are coming out to use their voice and to raise awareness."

On this point, Moutier added, in response to a question, that people in the field are seeing the use of language start to change. For example, after Anthony Bourdain's and Kate Spade's suicide deaths in June 2018, many more interviews with journalists started with requests to get the language right. "There's clearly a progression going on with regard to awareness about that. It doesn't mean they're always getting it right, of course, but there does seem to be movement in that regard."

Since 2006, continued Moutier, 32 states have passed laws mandating K–12 teacher training, and 18 states have enacted laws governing prevention and postvention in K–12 schools since 2012. States have also passed laws covering suicide prevention in health care training and in higher education. States have been calling for the enforcement of the federal law requiring parity for mental health benefits, and 13 federal laws have passed over the last decade involving suicide prevention.

As an example of how education of community and family members is occurring, Moutier briefly described the American Foundation for Suicide Prevention's Talk Saves Lives program, which has been delivered to tens of thousands of people in all 50 states. A sort of suicide prevention 101, the Talk Saves Lives program tells people that suicide is a health issue and that suicide can be prevented. It teaches people about the scope and epidemiology of suicide, about the risk factors demonstrated by research to drive up suicide risk, and about effective suicide prevention. The program teaches people about limiting access to lethal means through carbon dioxide sensors in cars, barriers on bridges, blister packaging for medications, firearm controls, and other means, especially during periods of risk. It disseminates educational materials at walks, health fairs, workplaces, and clinics. Examples of educational materials available from the American Foundation for Suicide Prevention include "After a Suicide Attempt," "Firearms and Suicide Prevention," and "After a Suicide."

This education effort, Moutier said, shows that everyone has a role to play in suicide prevention and culminates in the message that people should bring those who are at risk for suicide to a health care provider, "just as we want people to come to health care settings at the earliest indication that they might have diabetes or any other kind of health problem." Just as for other health problems, health care systems need to know what to do and deliver care for people at the earliest stages of deterioration in mental health or increase in suicide risk.

TREATMENT AS A PART OF SUICIDE PREVENTION

Moutier described several innovations in clinical treatments that are related to suicide prevention. First, several newly developed and evidence-based ways to reduce the risk of suicide are now available. For example, brief interventions are now being widely used, such as safety planning and lethal means counseling, that can be done during a single outpatient or emergency department visit. Treatments and peer support are now available online, and predictive analytics are being used to guide treatment and outreach. Such interventions have been shown to reduce the risk of suicide and need to be made much more accessible to the public, she said.

Health care systems need to consider suicide a health-related outcome and measure indicators related to suicide, she added. Critical windows exist for suicide risk, including the week after a psychiatric admission, the week after a psychiatric discharge, discharge from an emergency department following presentation for suicidal ideation or attempt, and the first weeks after starting an antidepressant (see Figure 2-5). Other periods of transition, such as a soldier transitioning to civilian status or a middle-aged man changing jobs or getting divorced, also have proven to be times of increased risk.

Several psychotherapies have been shown to reduce the risk of suicide; Moutier described two in detail. Dialectic behavioral therapy (DBT) has been evaluated in several landmark studies involving people with borderline personality disorder, substance use disorders, and eating disorders;

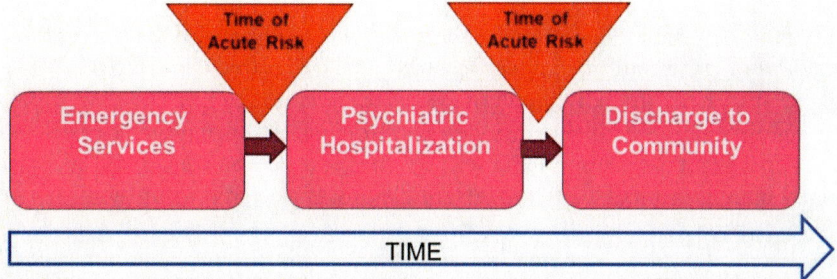

FIGURE 2-5 Transitions from one care setting to another can be periods of increased suicide risk.
SOURCES: Presented by Christine Moutier on September 11, 2018, at the Workshop on Improving Care to Prevent Suicide Among People with Serious Mental Illness. Used with permission from Elizabeth Ballard.

prepubescent children with disruptive mood dysregulation disorder; and adolescents with a suicide attempt history. For example, Linehan et al. (2006) conducted a randomized controlled trial of 101 women with borderline personality disorder who had recently attempted suicide. They were randomized into one of two groups and followed for 2 years. One group received DBT, while the other group received community expert therapy. The rate of reattempt was about 50 percent lower among the women who received DBT, and they had significantly fewer hospitalizations.

In a study of cognitive behavioral therapy (CBT), Brown et al. (2005) randomized 120 adults seen in an emergency department after a suicide attempt to either 10 sessions of CBT versus enhanced treatment as usual in the community. The study targeted the suicidal cognitions of these individuals, who were followed for 18 months. The participants who received CBT were 50 percent less likely to reattempt suicide than the usual care group, and their depression scores were significantly lower than the usual care group. "I want you to note that they had the same rate of suicidal ideation, so people can live with suicidal thoughts," said Moutier, adding:

> But the quality of their mental health and their behavior changed significantly. This is a new way to think about it. For many clinicians, we have not learned these things and have avoided honing in on our patient's suicidal thoughts. . . . This needs to start being incorporated as a part of treatment.

In a study of brief cognitive behavioral therapy, Rudd et al. (2015) customized CBT for a group of army soldiers who were either postsuicide attempt or had suicidal ideation with intent. Over a 2-year follow-up period, the group that received the brief CBT had a 60 percent lower risk of suicide attempts. On a larger scale, a meta-analysis of CBT targeted at suicidal ideations and behaviors found that the therapy was effective in five of six studies examined (Mewton and Andrews, 2016).

Moutier talked briefly about medications while noting that her discussion could not be comprehensive. She emphasized the need both to optimally manage primary psychiatric conditions, whether with medications or other approaches, and to incorporate considerations specific to suicide in treatment planning. A robust literature shows that lithium, compared with other mood stabilizers and other medications, and for both bipolar and unipolar mood disorders, reduces the risk of suicide attempts and death by suicide between 60 and 80 percent (Baldessarini et al., 2003, 2006), yet lithium is "a very underutilized medication." Clozapine is the only medication with a Food and Drug Administration (FDA) indication specific to suicide risk reduction for people with schizophrenia (Meltzer et al., 2003). With regard to antidepressants, the FDA black box warning has had the unintended consequence of confusing and alarming the public and leading to undertreatment of depressions among primary care doctors, Moutier said, but "there is a place for antidepressants in terms of risk reduction for suicide."

A newer class of medications, the NMDA blockers and related medications, has been given the "breakthrough therapy" designation by FDA because their efficacy data look so positive. For example, a single intravenous infusion of ketamine, a dissociative anesthetic from the 1960s, has shown evidence of an acute therapeutic effect for treatment-refractory depression (Muller et al., 2016). It also has produced a rapid reduction in suicidal ideation, starting in just a few hours and being sustained for about 1 week.

"That effect on reducing suicidal ideation has been shown to be partially independent of whether or not the mood effect occurs," said Moutier, "which is fascinating to separate out depression from suicidal ideation." The controversy around ketamine relates to the small size of most studies, the potential for abuse, potential side effects such as dissociation, and the relatively short length of therapeutic effect. Other medications similar to Ketamine, such as esketamine and rapastinel, are in the pipeline.

PROJECT 2025

Several years ago, a group of organizations, including the Substance Abuse and Mental Health Services Administration, the National Institute of Mental Health, the National Action Alliance for Suicide Prevention, and CDC, joined the American Foundation for Suicide Prevention in setting a goal of reducing the annual suicide rate in the United States 20 percent by 2025. Informed by an American Foundation for Suicide Prevention expert panel thorough analysis of the research literature, and using a system dynamic model to project potential lives saved, they are taking four pathways toward the goal. The first was to infuse suicide prevention education into communities that own firearms. The second was to change practices in emergency departments, because 39 percent of people make an emergency department visit in the year prior to a suicide and 70 percent do not attend the first outpatient appointment after an attempt. The third was to work with health care systems, because up to 45 percent of individuals who die by suicide visit their primary care physician in the month prior. The fourth was to focus on corrections systems, because suicide accounts for 35 percent of all deaths in jails.

Project 2025 takes an evidence-based, pragmatic approach to reducing the national suicide rate. Many other organizations have now joined in this project, including accrediting bodies, trade organizations, and professional organizations, Moutier observed. These organizations can recommend, suggest, mandate, and set new standards to significantly reduce the suicide rate.

CLOSING THE GAPS

Finally, Moutier discussed some of the gaps in suicide prevention and ways of filling those gaps. She noted that federal investments in research in such leading causes of death as HIV/AIDS, heart disease, and prostate cancer have led to substantial declines in the death rate from those conditions (see Figure 2-6). For suicide, however, federal investments have been "rather meager," she observed, and the suicide rate is continuing to climb.

Another gap has, until recently, been standards of care in clinical practice for people at risk for suicide. The publication by the National Action Alliance for Suicide Prevention (2018) of a recommended standard care for people with suicide risk has helped meet this need.

Other gaps described by Moutier include the need to achieve universal mental health literacy so that people know what to do well upstream of suicide risk becoming apparent, implementation science to measure the effect of clinical treatments and community-based programs, inclusion rather than exclusion of people at risk for suicide in clinical trials, better surveillance and health systems to capture data about suicide-related events and deaths, clinician training in prevention, integrated mental health care and screening in primary care, the ability to bill for services such as lethal means counseling or peer-to-peer and telemedicine services, and enforcement of mental health parity.

"By doing all of these things together, we can save lives and improve the quality of many more," said Moutier. "We are gaining traction in creating a culture that is much more savvy about mental health and suicide prevention, and that's a wonderful thing."

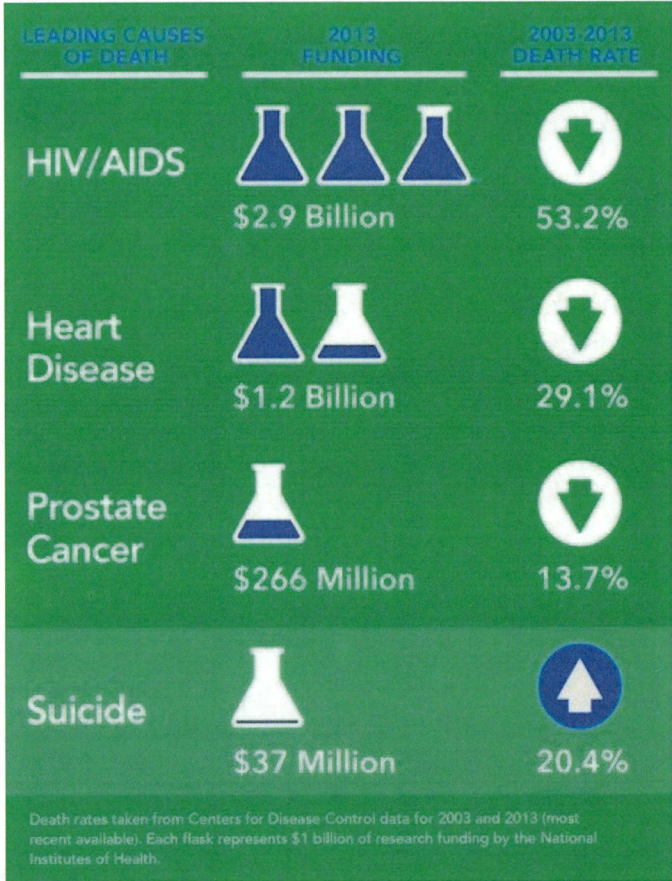

FIGURE 2-6 Suicide prevention has received little federal funding even as suicide rates have risen.
NOTE: HIV/AIDS = human immunodeficiency virus/acquired immunodeficiency syndrome.
SOURCES: Presented by Christine Moutier on September 11, 2018, at the Workshop on Improving Care to Prevent Suicide Among People with Serious Mental Illness. From American Foundation for Suicide Prevention.

THE EFFECTS OF SCREENING

In response to a question about screening for suicide during primary care visits, Moutier discussed data from the Emergency Department Safety Assessment and Follow-up Evaluation (ED-SAFE) study, which sought to apply universal screening to the extent possible in emergency departments. Screening approximately doubled the identification of patients in eight emergency departments who were having current suicidal ideation or had a recent suicide attempt. "Certainly our first step is to identify those patients who are at risk and then of course to apply the appropriate care steps."

Wilcox added that suicide risk screening has gained momentum with the Joint Commission encouraging hospitals to detect suicidal ideation through screening. Screening is not able to catch everyone at risk at the right time. "That being said, I find from my experience it to be useful, because . . . multiple studies are showing converging evidence that screening can substantially increase detection."

On this point, Michael Schoenbaum, senior advisor for mental health services, epidemiology, and economics in the Division of Services and Intervention Research at the National Institute of Mental Health, observed that the best evidence for the efficacy of screening occurs not in general wellness or outpatient primary care settings but in emergency care settings, as in the ED-SAFE study. He also noted that the ED-SAFE study had a phase in which it did universal screening but did not enhance care for the people identified, which revealed that screening by itself did not change the subsequent suicide risk outcomes. Screening needs to be followed by safety planning and follow-up contact after discharge to be effective, he said. The ED-SAFE study also found that patients who were identified through screening and patients who volunteered the information that they had suicidal ideation or had physical problems that indicated self-harm were statistically indistinguishable in terms of their subsequent risk. In other words, the people who are being identified through screening are "not just answering the question lightly because somebody asked them. They're the people you need to be looking for."

PERSONAL INTERVENTIONS

Linda Beeber, president of the board of directors for the American Psychiatric Nurses Association and Francis Hill Fox Distinguished Term Professor at the University of North Carolina at Chapel Hill School of Nursing, noted that the association is equipping 12,000 nurses with scripts and slide sets to educate their communities about such subjects as mental health, violence, and suicide; it also is reaching out to the 3 million registered nurses to increase their mental health literacy. But what about educating the general public about suicide prevention, she asked.

Moutier responded that the American Foundation for Suicide Prevention has scripted a series of steps for having a caring conversation. "It's as simple as the type of caring conversation you would have with anyone in your life that you're worried about for any reason." The script calls for explaining that you are there to support a person and not to pass judgment. For a parent, it is important to say that no challenge a child is facing will change the way they feel about their child. "That expression of unconditional love is something that we often assume, and sometimes our behavior doesn't always stay consistent, so we need to say it in that moment." The script then addresses suicidal ideation and knowing where 24/7 resources are and how to access them. She also noted that suicidal ideation is a common phenomenon. "We don't necessarily need to bring everyone who's having suicidal thoughts straight to the ER. Many people are living with that." Providing that understanding to people is part of deepening mental health literacy. But exactly what to do and when to do it can be challenging, Moutier said.

She also mentioned an ad campaign launched by the Ad Council, the American Foundation for Suicide Prevention, and the Jed Foundation called Seize the Awkward that targets 16- to 24-year-olds who are concerned about a friend but do not know how to reach out.[1] "There's a whole toolkit around how to start the conversation, how to continue the conversation, how to come back to it, [how not to] take it personally if they rebuff you." In response to a related question, she also noted that social media and broadcast media can spread awareness:

> We work with anyone who will work with us in the industry, including some major media people who have become interested. Accurate, safe, and effective messaging can save lives, so partnering with media and entertainment industry leaders is key. It just requires relationship development, trust, and empathy to understand the challenges that they're facing.

COVERAGE, DIGITAL TECHNOLOGIES, AND PHYSICIAN CARE

In response to a question about covering peer-support services under Medicare, Wilcox praised the peer-support model, though she noted that issues continue to surround how best to train and support peers, especially if they are in recovery. "These are all things that hopefully will be sorted out as we move more toward implementing that model in communities." Beeber from the American Psychiatric Nurses Association added that she is on the congressionally mandated Interdepartmental Serious Mental Illness Coordinating Committee, which has been examining the issue of Medicare coverage for peer support, and that the issue has come up and will continue to be pursued.

In response to a question about digital health technologies, Moutier said that advances in this area require truly interdisciplinary science. "It's a new kind of way to do science, and investments clearly could be utilized to motivate more of those disciplines to come together. It's already happening, but much more needs to happen." An example is the Resources for Enhancing Alzheimer's Caregivers Health Veterans Affairs (REACH VA) program

---

[1] The campaign can be found at https://seizetheawkward.org (accessed November 27, 2018).

at the Veterans Health Administration, which is using data analytics to analyze 100 data points in electronic health records and using that information to actively reach out to veterans. "Once we know more about how that's going, we can learn from that," Moutier said. Wilcox, too, pointed to the benefits of being able to use data in real time for intervention. It can take years to get suicide data, making it difficult to use data for action. One option, she said, is to use social media data for targeted interventions, which is "an area of great promise for the future."

With regard to integrated data systems, Moutier noted that the Zero Suicide program is building a system that is integrated in such a way as to pay attention to all the data points that indicate suicide risk. Then people are trained to respond to that information and to make sure that patients do not fall through the cracks. Wilcox added that one complication involves data coding for predictive analytics. Important data often reside in the notes, but these typically are not coded. Work in such areas as natural language processing may be able to overcome this problem, "but it's a complex issue that's going to take some time to get all the technology sorted out to be able to do this in a large scale." In particular, issues of privacy and data protection are major concerns in this area.

Finally, a question about preventing suicide among physicians led Moutier to respond "thanks for bringing my passion area up." Physicians live in a culture where seeking help has been stigmatized and mental health has been erroneously equated with impairment. But change is happening at both the system and local levels. For example, the American Council for Graduate Medical Education now requires that all residency training programs in the United States have programs for wellness and access to 24/7 mental health support for residents. "There's been a radical shift over the last about 4 years in academic medicine," Moutier said.

REFERENCES

Anglemyer, A., T. Horvath, and G. Rutherford. 2014. The accessibility of firearms and risk for suicide and homicide victimization among household members: A systematic review and meta-analysis. *Annals of Internal Medicine* 160(2):101-110.

Baldessarini, R. J., L. Tondo, and J. Hennen. 2003. Lithium treatment and suicide risk in major affective disorders: Update and new findings. *Journal of Clinical Psychiatry* 64(Suppl 5):44-52.

Baldessarini, R. J., L. Tondo, P. Davis, M. Pompili, F. K. Goodwin, and J. Hennen. 2006. Decreased risk of suicides and attempts during long-term lithium treatment: A meta-analytic review. *Bipolar Disorders* 8(5 Pt 2):625-639.

Bastiampillai, T., S. S. Sharfstein, and S. Allison. 2016. Increase in US suicide rates and the critical decline in psychiatric beds. *JAMA* 316(24):2591-2592.

Bilukha, O., R. A. Hahn, A. Crosby, M. T. Fullilove, A. Liberman, E. Moscicki, S. Snyder, F. Tuma, P. Corso, A. Schofield, P. A. Briss, and the Task Force on Community Preventive Services. 2005. The effectiveness of early childhood home visitation in preventing violence: A systematic review. *American Journal of Preventive Medicine* 28(2 Suppl 1):11-39.

Bolton, J. M., and J. Robinson. 2010. Population-attributable fractions of Axis I and Axis II mental disorders for suicide attempts: Findings from a representative sample of the adult, noninstitutionalized U.S. population. *American Journal of Public Health* 100(12):2473-2480.

Brown, G. K., T. Ten Have, G. R. Henriques, S. X. Xie, J. E. Hollander, and A. T. Beck. 2005. Cognitive therapy for the prevention of suicide attempts: A randomized controlled trial. *Journal of the American Medical Association* 294(5):563-570.

Case, A., and A. Deaton. 2017. Mortality and Morbidity in the 21st century. *Brookings Papers on Economic Activity* Spring 397-476.

Cavanagh, J. T., A. J. Carson, M. Sharpe, and S. M. Lawrie. 2003. Psychological autopsy studies of suicide: A systematic review. *Psychological Medicine* 33(3):395-405.

Connell, A. M., H. N. McKillop, and T. J. Dishion. 2016. Long-term effects of the family check-up in early adolescence on risk of suicide in early adulthood. *Suicide and Life-Threatening Behavior* 46(Suppl 1):S15-S22.

Crifasi, C. K., J. S. Meyers, J. S. Vernick, and D. W. Webster. 2015. Effects of changes in permit-to-purchase handgun laws in Connecticut and Missouri on suicide rates. *Preventive Medicine* 79:43-49.

Cwik, M. F., L. Tingey, A. Maschino, N. Goklish, F. Larzelere-Hinton, J. Walkup, and A. Barlow. 2016. Decreases in suicide deaths and attempts linked to the White Mountain Apache Suicide Surveillance and Prevention System, 2001-2012. *American Journal of Public Health* 106(12):2183-2189.

Franklin, J. C., J. D. Ribeiro, K. R. Fox, K. H. Bentley, E. M. Kleiman, X. Huang, K. M. Musacchio, A. C. Jaroszewski, B. P. Chang, and M. K. Nock. 2017. Risk factors for suicidal thoughts and behaviors: A meta-analysis of 50 years of research. *Psychological Bulletin* 143(2):187-232.

Hahn, R. A., O. O. Bilukha, A. Crosby, M. T. Fullilove, A. Liberman, E. K. Moscicki, S. Snyder, F. Tuma, A. Schofield, P. S. Corso, P. Briss, and Task Force on Community Preventive Services. 2003. First reports evaluating the effectiveness of strategies for preventing violence: Early childhood home visitation. Findings from the Task Force on Community Preventive Services. *Morbidity and Mortality Weekly Report* 52(RR-14):1-9.

Halla, M. 2013. The effect of joint custody on family outcomes. *Journal of the European Economic Association* 11(2):278-315.

Hawkins, J. S., R. Kosterman, R. F. Catalano, K. G. Hill, and R. D. Abbott. 2005. Promoting positive adult functioning through social development intervention in childhood: Long-term effects from the Seattle Social Development Project. *Archives of Pediatrics and Adolescent Medicine* 159(1):25-31.

Kellermann, A. L., F. P. Rivara, G. Somes, D. T. Reay, J. Francisco, J. G. Banton, J. Prodzinski, C. Fligner, and B. B. Hackman. 1992. Suicide in the home in relation to gun ownership. *New England Journal of Medicine* 327(7):467-472.

Kessler, R. C., C. H. Warner, C. Ivany, M. V. Petukhova, S. Rose, E. J. Bromet, M. Brown 3rd, T. Cai, L. J. Colpe, K. L. Cox, C. S. Fullerton, S. E. Gilman, M. J. Gruber, S. G. Heeringa, L. Lewandowski-Romps, J. Li, A. M. Millikan-Bell, J. A. Naifeh, M. K. Nock, A. J. Rosellini, N. A. Sampson, M. Schoenbaum, M. B. Stein, S. Wessely, A. M. Zaslavsky, R. J. Ursano, and the Army STARRS Collaborators. 2015. Predicting suicides after psychiatric hospitalization in U.S. Army soldiers: The Army Study To Assess Risk and Resilience in Servicemembers (Army STARRS). *Journal of the American Medical Association Psychiatry* 72(1):49-57.

Knox, K. L., D. A. Lotts, G. W. Talcott, J. C. Feig, and E. D Caine. 2003. Risk of suicide and related adverse outcomes after exposure to a suicide prevention programme in the U.S. Air Force: Cohort study. *BMJ* 327(7428):1376.
Knox, K. L., S. Pflanz, G. W. Talcott, R. L. Campise, J. E. Lavigne, A. Bajorska, X. Tu, and E. D. Caine. 2010. The U.S. Air Force suicide prevention program: Implications for public health policy. *American Journal of Public Health* 100(12):2457-2463.
Linehan, M. M., K. A. Comtois, A. M. Murray, M. Z. Brown, R. J. Gallop, H. L. Heard, K. E. Korslund, D. A. Tutek, S. K. Reynolds, and N. Lindenboim. 2006. Two-year randomized controlled trial and follow-up of dialectical behavior therapy vs therapy by experts for suicidal behaviors and borderline personality disorder. *Archives of General Psychiatry* 63(7):757-766.
March, J. S., B. J. Klee, and C. M. Kremer. 2006. Treatment benefit and the risk of suicidality in multicenter, randomized, controlled trials of sertraline in children and adolescents. *Journal of Child and Adolescent Psychopharmacology* 16(1-2):91-102.
McCarthy, J. F., M. Valenstein, H. M. Kim, M. Ilgen, K. Zivin, and F. C. Blow. 2009. Suicide mortality among patients receiving care in the Veterans Health Administration health system. *American Journal of Epidemiology* 169(8):1033-1038.
McCarthy, J. F., R. M. Bossarte, I. R. Katz, C. Thompson, J. Kemp, C. M. Hannemann, C. Nielson, and M. Schoenbaum. 2015. Predictive modeling and concentration of the risk of suicide: Implications for preventive interventions in the U.S. Department of Veterans Affairs. *American Journal of Public Health* 105(9):1935-1942.
Meltzer, H. Y., L. Alphs, A. I. Green, A. C. Altamura, R. Anand, A. Bertoldi, M. Bourgeois, G. Chouinard, M. Z. Islam, J. Kane, R. Krishnan, J. P. Lindenmayer, S. Potkin, and the International Suicide Prevention Trial Study Group. 2003. Clozapine treatment for suicidality in schizophrenia: International Suicide Prevention Trial (InterSePT). *Archives of General Psychiatry* 60(1):82-91.
Mewton, L., and G. Andrews. 2016. Cognitive behavioral therapy for suicidal behaviors: Improving patient outcomes. *Psychology Research and Behavior Management* 9:21-29.
Miller, M., and D. Hemenway. 2008. Guns and suicide in the United States. *New England Journal of Medicine* 359(10):989-991.
Miller, M., C. Barber, R. A. White, and D. Azrael. 2013. Firearms and suicide in the United States: Is risk independent of underlying suicidal behavior? *American Journal of Epidemiology* 178(6):946-955.
Muller, J., S. Pentyala, J. Dilger, and S. Pentyala S. 2016. Ketamine enantiomers in the rapid and sustained antidepressant effects. *Therapeutic Advances in Psychopharmacology* 6(3):185-192.
National Action Alliance for Suicide Prevention: Transforming Health Systems Initiative Work Group. 2018. *Recommended standard care for people with suicide risk: Making health care suicide safe*. Washington, DC: Education Development Center, Inc.
Nock, M. K., A. J. Millner, P. M. Gutierrez, J. A. Naifeh, M. B. Stein, R. C. Kessler, T. E. Joiner, G. Han, I. Hwang, A. King, N. A. Sampson, A. M. Zaslavsky, and R. J. Ursano. 2018. Risk factors for the transition from suicide ideation to suicide attempt: Results from the Army Study to Assess Risk and Resilience in Servicemembers (Army STARRS). *Journal of Abnormal Psychology* 127(2):139-149. https://nocklab.fas.harvard.edu/files/nocklab/files/29528668-nock-2018.pdf (accessed December 5, 2018).
Rudd, M. D., C. J. Bryan, E. G. Wertenberger, A. L. Peterson, S. Young-McCaughan, J. Mintz, S. R. Williams, K. A. Arne, J. Breitbach, K. Delano, E. Wilkinson, and T. O. Bruce. 2015. Brief cognitive-behavioral therapy effects on post-treatment suicide attempts in a military sample: Results of a randomized clinical trial with 2-year follow-up. *American Journal of Psychiatry* 172(5):441-449.

Shepard, D. S., D. Gurewich, A. K. Lwin, G. A. Reed, Jr., and M. M. Silverman. 2016. Suicide and suicidal attempts in the United States: Costs and policy implications. *Suicide and Life-Threatening Behavior* 46(3):352-362.

Simon, G. E., E. Johnson, J. M. Lawrence, R. C. Rossom, B. Ahmedani, F. L. Lynch, A. Beck, B. Waitzfelder, R. Ziebell, R. B. Penfold, and S. M. Shortreed. 2018. Predicting suicide attempts and suicide deaths following outpatient visits using electronic health records. *American Journal of Psychiatry* 175(10):951-960.

Stevenson, B., and J. Wolfers. 2006. Bargaining in the shadow of the law: Divorce laws and family distress. *Quarterly Journal of Economics* 121(1):267-288.

Stone, D. M., T. R. Simon, K. A. Fowler, S. R. Kegler, K. Yuan, K. M. Holland, A. Z. Ivey-Stephenson, and A. E. Crosby. 2018. Vital signs: Trends in state suicide rates—United States, 1999-2016 and circumstances contributing to suicide—27 States, 2015. *Morbidity and Mortality Weekly Report* 67(22):617-624.

Tidemalm, D., N. Långström, P. Lichtenstein, and B. Runeson. 2008. Risk of suicide after suicide attempt according to coexisting psychiatric disorder: Swedish cohort study with long term follow-up. *BMJ* 337:a2205.

Tran, T., W. Luo, D. Phung, R. Harvey, M. Berk, R. L. Kennedy, and S. Venkatesh. 2014. Risk stratification using data from electronic medical records better predicts suicide risks than clinician assessments. 2014. *BMC Psychiatry* 14:76.

Wasserman, D., C. W. Hoven, C. Wasserman, M. Wall, R. Eisenberg, G. Hadlaczky, I. Kelleher, M. Sarchiapone, A. Apter, J. Balazs, J. Bobes, R. Brunner, P. Corcoran, D. Cosman, F. Guillemin, C. Haring, M. Iosue, M. Kaess, J. P. Kahn, H. Keeley, G. J. Musa, B. Nemes, V. Postuvan, P. Saiz, S. Reiter-Theil, A. Varnik, P. Varnik, and V. Carli. 2015. School-based suicide prevention programmes: The SEYLE cluster-randomised, controlled trial. *Lancet* 385(9977):1536-1544.

While, D., H. Bickley, A. Roscoe, K. Windfuhr, S. Rahman, J. Shaw, L. Appleby, and N. Kapur. 2012. Implementation of mental health service recommendations in England and Wales and suicide rates, 1997-2006: A cross-section and before-and-after observational study. *Lancet* 379:1005-1012.

Wilcox, H. C., S. G. Kellam, C. H. Brown, J. M. Poduska, N. S. Ialongo, W. Wang, and J. C. Anthony. 2008. The impact of two universal randomized first- and second-grade classroom interventions on young adult suicide ideation and attempts. *Drug and Alcohol Dependence* 95(Suppl 1):S60-S73.

Wintemute, G. J. 2015. Alcohol misuse, firearm violence perpetration, and public policy in the United States. *Preventive Medicine* 79:15-21.

Wolk, C. B., P. C. Kendall, and R. S. Beidas. 2015. Cognitive-behavioral therapy for child anxiety confers long-term protection from suicidality. *Journal of the American Academy of Child and Adolescent Psychiatry* 54(3):175-179.

3

Suicide Prevention in Health Care Systems

> **Points Made by the Presenters**
>
> - Health care settings provide an important opportunity to intervene for suicide prevention. (Hogan)
> - Evidence for the effectiveness of suicide-focused care demonstrates that, for those with serious mental illness and risk of suicide, interventions for mental illness are important but not sufficient. Integrated care that treats both the underlying mental disorder and suicidality is more likely to be more effective. (Hogan)
> - The Perfect Depression Care Initiative and its goal of zero suicide dramatically reduced suicide rates at the Henry Ford Health System and provided a proof-of-concept model that other systems have adopted. (E. Coffey)
> - The Zero Suicide model is a comprehensive evidence-based approach to improving health care quality that has three essential components: the conviction that ideal health care is attainable, a road map to achieve that vision, and a requisite expertise in systems engineering to achieve the vision. (E. Coffey)
> - A standard protocol for managing suicide risk in health care settings can ensure that people with suicidality do not make their way through successive potential gaps in care: asking people about suicide, providing a safety planning intervention,

reducing lethal means, treating suicidality, and ensuring that interpersonal, structured support is available. (Hogan)
- Suicide prevention activities have previously been out of scope for health care; health care and behavioral health professionals have not received training on them; and securing reimbursement for these activities takes works. Leadership is needed for health care to adopt these responsibilities. (Hogan)
- Suicide is a worldwide problem that requires a worldwide response. (Covington)

NOTE: These points were made by the individual workshop presenters identified above. They are not intended to reflect a consensus among workshop participants.

During the second panel of the workshop, three presenters talked about major initiatives in health care systems that have had major effects on suicide rates. These initiatives point toward the possibility of making much more extensive changes in health care systems, both in the United States and abroad, that could achieve for suicide prevention the successes achieved through prevention initiatives targeting health issues such as smoking or heart disease.

THE ORIGIN OF THE ZERO SUICIDE MODEL

In 2001 the Institute of Medicine (IOM) released the report *Crossing the Quality Chasm: A New Health System for the 21st Century* (IOM, 2001). As C. Edward Coffey, professor of psychiatry and behavioral sciences and of neurology in the Baylor College of Medicine, recounted, the report observed that health care providers are well trained, are working as hard as they can, and are trying to do the right thing. But, as the report stated,

> In its current form, habits, and environment, the health care system is incapable of giving Americans the health care they want and deserve. . . . The current care systems cannot do the job. Trying harder will not work. Changing systems of care will.

The report laid out six dimensions of ideal care. Such care is:

- Safe,
- Effective,
- Patient-centered,

- Timely,
- Efficient, and
- Equitable.

The report also provided 10 rules for designing a system that would achieve ideal care:

- Care equals relationships.
- Care is customized.
- Care is patient-centered.
- Share knowledge.
- Manage by fact.
- Make safety a system priority.
- Embrace transparency.
- Anticipate patient needs.
- Continually reduce waste.
- Professionals cooperate.

After the report was published, the Robert Wood Johnson Foundation (RWJF) partnered with the Institute for Healthcare Improvement (IHI) to launch the RWJF Pursuing Perfection Program, which had as its goal to demonstrate that ideal health care is attainable. Using the IOM report as a guide, the foundation sought applications for transformative plans to create health care systems that would approach ideal care within a timeframe of 2 years. From about 300 applications submitted in 2001, 12 finalists were selected, including the Perfect Depression Care Initiative proposed by the Behavioral Health Services Division of Henry Ford Health System in Detroit, Michigan. "We celebrated for about 10 seconds," said E. Coffey, who was then chief executive officer of behavioral health services for the system and the principal investigator on the Perfect Depression Care Initiative. "Then we started thinking, what in the world are we going to do to try to transform our mental health care system?"

The finalists were required to develop "perfection" goals for each of the six dimensions of ideal care. The Henry Ford Perfect Depression Care Initiative accordingly established the following goals (Coffey, 2006, 2007):

- Safe care: Eliminate inpatient falls and medication errors.
- Effective care: Eliminate suicides.
- Patient-centered care: 100 percent of patients will be completely satisfied with their care.
- Timely care: 100 percent complete satisfaction.
- Efficient care: 100 percent complete satisfaction.
- Equitable care: 100 percent complete satisfaction.

The goal for effective care was initially unclear until a staff member, in one of the many meetings held to discuss the goals, said, "Well, perhaps if we were doing perfect depression care, nobody would die from suicide. Nobody would kill themselves." Recounted E. Coffey: "At that moment, after we all got our breath back, our department was transformed.... That moment, essentially, was the birth of Zero Suicide."

With zero suicides becoming the overarching goal, E. Coffey's group adapted a planned care model designed to create productive interactions (see Figure 3-1). These interactions result from an informed and activated patient working closely with a prepared and proactive practice team. The elements of these interactions correspond closely with the goals of the IOM report.

During the first decade of the 21st century, the suicide rate was increasing in Michigan. However, after implementation of the Perfect Depression Care Initiative, the suicide rate for patients receiving mental health care in the Henry Ford Health System dropped by more than 75 percent, though the rate rose again in 2010 when the recession that began in 2008 was especially severe in Michigan (Coffey et al., 2015). In most years, the suicide rate for the system was close to that of the general population in Michigan, even though the expected suicide rate for people with an active mood disorder is approximately 21 times the rate for the general population, E. Coffey observed.

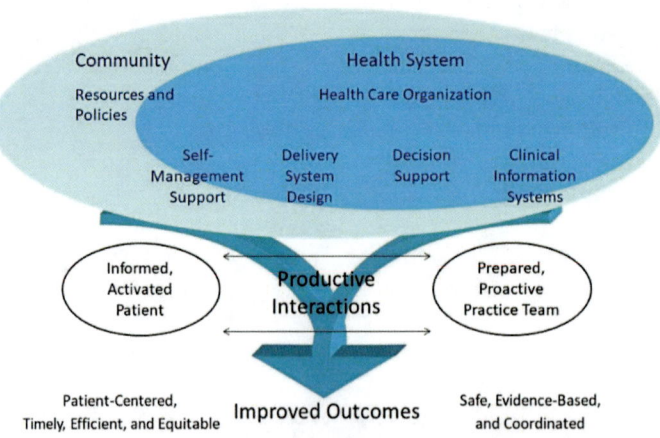

FIGURE 3-1 The planned care model implemented by the Henry Ford Health System.
SOURCE: Presented by C. Edward Coffey on September 11, 2018, at the Workshop on Improving Care to Prevent Suicide Among People with Serious Mental Illness.

E. Coffey emphasized that depression is not the only risk factor for suicide. All the major mental disorders raise the risk of suicide, especially if they are comorbid with substance use disorder. "If you're trying to bend the curve on suicide risk, you don't want to focus just on depression." They therefore worked to ensure that all their patients received "perfect" care.

Improvement projects are not complete until their results have been described and disseminated, noted E. Coffey. To address this need, the Perfect Depression Care team produced a series of articles describing the initiative and its results over time (Coffey, 2006, 2007; Hampton, 2010; Ahmedani et al., 2013; Coffey et al., 2013; Coffey and Coffey, 2016). The public feedback was very positive, including recognition as a best-in-class innovation by the Malcolm Baldrige examiners when they awarded the Henry Ford Health System the 2011 Malcolm Baldrige National Quality Award. In 2012 the Perfect Depression Care Initiative was invited by Mike Hogan and David Covington to partner with the National Action Alliance for Suicide Prevention, a partnership which has yielded a "hugely productive" collaboration that has embraced the goal of Zero Suicide (see the following section of this chapter). Other organizations, including the National Institute of Mental Health and the Centers for Disease Control and Prevention (CDC), have subsequently embraced the goals of the Zero Suicide model. International Zero Suicide summits beginning in 2014 have provided a way to exchange information and spread the program to other health care systems (see "International Actions on Suicide Prevention" later in this chapter). Early adopters of the Zero Suicide model have included an organization in Tennessee known as Centerstone, as well as the National Health Service, the Mersey Care Trust, and Zero Suicide Alliance, all in the United Kingdom.

Such initiatives are desperately needed, said E. Coffey. As pointed out earlier in the workshop by Wilcox and Moutier, suicide rates have increased 30 percent over the past 15 years, with an even greater increase in some states (see Figure 3-2). "Despite all the great work that is being done, and all the great progress scientifically, and even despite Zero Suicide, the curve is moving in the wrong direction in this country." A possible explanation for this discrepancy may lie in the distinction between zero suicide as an aspirational goal versus Zero Suicide as a firm goal that serves as an innovative driving force for transformation to ideal health care (Coffey, 2003). As an innovation, the Zero Suicide model has three key elements. The first is a radical new conviction that ideal health care is attainable. The second is a road map to achieve that vision ("pursuing perfection within a just culture"). The third is expertise in systems engineering to implement the vision.

The challenge today, said E. Coffey, is that Zero Suicide may be seen as a stand-alone aspirational goal rather than as an essential component in this tripartite model of transformation. "I don't want to complain about

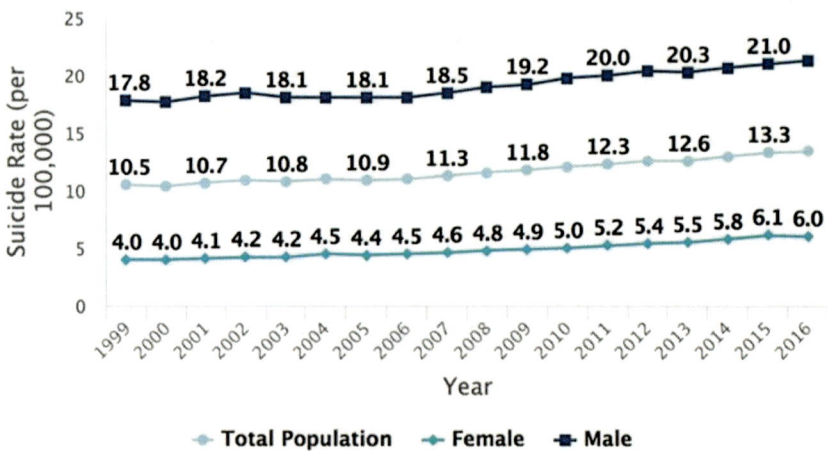

FIGURE 3-2 Age-adjusted suicide rates rose 30 percent in the United States between 1999 and 2016.
SOURCES: Presented by C. Edward Coffey on September 11, 2018, at the Workshop on Improving Care to Prevent Suicide Among People with Serious Mental Illness. From CDC, 2018.

any goal" that seeks to lower the suicide rate, he said, and a goal to reduce suicides by 20 percent before 2025 is great and should be encouraged. "But it may be that as long as we view Zero Suicide as an aspiration, we are backing away from being 'all in,' from being convinced that ideal health care is possible." Experience with Perfect Depression Care suggests that audacious goals such as "Zero Suicide" are essential components in driving transformation, said E. Coffey, and that transformation rather than incremental improvement is what is needed to bend the curve on suicide and give patients the care they want and deserve.

DISSEMINATION AND EVIDENCE FOR ZERO SUICIDE

Even as the suicide rate has increased in the past 15 years, the age-adjusted death rates for heart disease, cancer, and stroke have fallen. Why has prevention for other causes of death been successful while suicide prevention has not been successful, asked Mike Hogan of Hogan Health Solutions.

With deaths from cardiovascular disease (CVD), the reduction in smoking accounts for 20 to 25 percent of the improvement. However, targeted preventive interventions with people who have well-established CVD risks had an even greater effect. The Zero Suicide movement seeks to establish suicide prevention as a goal and a priority in health care. The model, like the successful efforts to reduce CVD deaths, emphasizes effective preventive interventions for those with elevated risk. But the health care system has not yet taken that goal to heart, Hogan said. Even in hospitals, a recent analysis found that the estimated number of inpatient deaths by suicide that occur each year ranges from 49 to 65 (Williams et al., 2018).

The Zero Suicide movement is also a care innovation, Hogan observed. It combines a quality improvement with a bundling of care, as has been the case with innovations applied to other health conditions. This point is made in the report *Suicide Care in Systems Framework* (Clinical Care and Intervention Task Force and National Action Alliance for Suicide Prevention, 2011), which looked at the applicability of the Henry Ford initiative in the larger health care system.

Research has shown that suicidal behavior is distinct from mental disorders (Van Orden et al., 2010). Many people have suicidal thoughts, but relatively few progress to attempts (Millner et al., 2017; Klonsky et al., 2018). "For the average person [in the Millner et al. study], it was 2 years between ideation and attempt," observed Hogan. "That's a lot of time to intervene, but only if we know. And since we tend to not ask, we don't know." However, once people have reached a tipping point, the time to an attempt was short—from a few minutes to a few weeks. Developing the "capability" to kill oneself is the dangerous step, said Hogan—both the internal capability and the physical capability to act. In addition, no single pathway from ideation to suicide exists. "Life is complicated, genetics are complicated, genetic–environmental interactions are complicated."

Health care settings provide places to intervene. First, more than 80 percent of people dying by suicide and more than 90 percent with attempts had health care visits in the previous 12 months. Of people who died from suicide, 45 percent had a primary care visit in the month before death, 19 percent had contact with mental health services in the month before, and 10 percent had an emergency department visit in the previous 60 days. The rates are even higher for older men, with 70 percent seeing a general practitioner within 30 days of a death by suicide. The risk of suicide death following inpatient psychiatric discharge is 44 times the population rate, observed Hogan. In short, the health care system has ample time to intervene. The question is whether it does.

The second reason why suicide prevention in health care settings makes sense, said Hogan, is that evidence exists for effective—often brief—interventions that can be deployed feasibly in health care organizations. Hogan presented a mental model that is used by Zero Suicide to illustrate how people who die by suicide fall through successive gaps in the health care system (see Figure 3-3). The first gap, said Hogan, is whether people are asked about suicide. The second is whether health care providers engage and provide a safety planning intervention to give people the skill set and

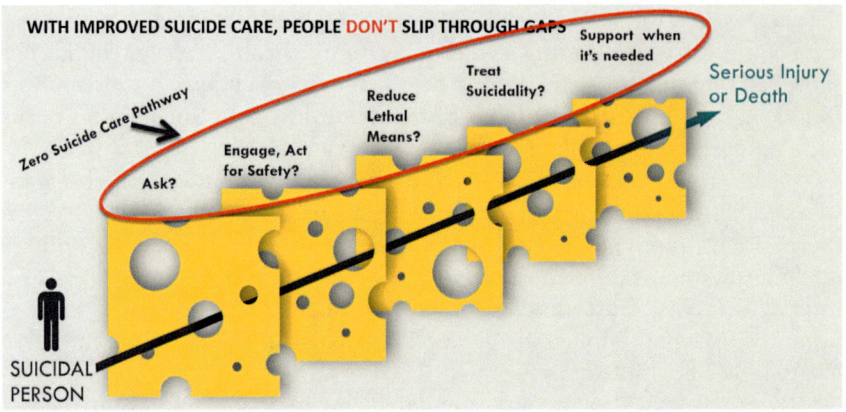

FIGURE 3-3 Improved care can keep people with suicidality from slipping through successive gaps in the health care system.
SOURCES: Presented by Mike Hogan on September 11, 2018, at the Workshop on Improving Care to Prevent Suicide Among People with Serious Mental Illness. From Zero Suicide Institute, Education Development Center, 2018.

tools they need. Successive steps involve reducing lethal means, treating suicidality, and ensuring that interpersonal, structured support is available when needed. "These actions need to be done in a routine way within a health care setting," said Hogan. "It's a care pathway. Not doing this would be the equivalent of having people in care for diabetes and never getting an A1C level."

Simon et al. (2013) examined the subsequent history of more than 75,000 people who completed the Patient Health Questionnaire 9 to screen for depression. Of those who subsequently died by suicide, 60 percent indicated elevated thoughts on question 9, which asks about "thoughts that you would be better off dead or hurting yourself in some way." The suicide field has had a debate about whether it is possible to predict who is going to die, and "we shouldn't be interested in predicting who's going to die," observed Hogan. "We should want to know who needs help. Cardiologists are not worried about [whether they can] predict when people are going to die of a heart attack and who that's going to be. They identify risk factors and then they take action." Based on the Simon et al. (2013) study, prediction of who needs suicide prevention are much better then high cholesterol scores are to predict a heart attack, Hogan said. "This is good enough evidence to act."

Safety planning makes sense, is feasible, and has become widely used, but until recently it had not been well tested, said Hogan. However, Stanley et al. (2018) recently did an emergency department matched cohort comparison study with 1,640 patients with a suicide-related visit and 1,186 in the intervention group. They tested a brief safety planning intervention plus telephone follow-up and found that the patients receiving the intervention had 45 percent fewer suicidal behaviors and were twice as likely to participate in follow-up care.

Means restriction is a critical part of a safety plan, and evidence and experience at a population level indicates that it works, said Hogan. In communities with a dominant means of suicide, restricting that means reduced suicide rates by about 40 percent. In addition, caring contacts, including phone calls, letters, texts, postcards, and visits, are effective. Denchev et al. (2018) found that caring letters work better than usual care and cost less, phone calls work even better, and cognitive behavioral therapy is also effective.

Evidence for the effectiveness of suicide-focused therapies over usual care comes from dialectical behavior therapy, cognitive therapy for suicide prevention, collaborative Assessment and Management of Suicide (CAMS), post-attempt counseling (from Denmark), and the Attempted Suicide Short Intervention Program (from Switzerland). This evidence from randomized controlled trials demonstrates that such therapies are as effective as acute care interventions for cardiovascular disease, said Hogan. The idea of directly treating suicidality is "fundamentally relevant" to the workshop, he observed. "If somebody is suicidal and has a major mental illness, it's no longer acceptable to just treat the major mental illness and hope that the suicidality resolves."

The critical issue, said Hogan, is that the usual care for people at risk of suicide is unacceptably bad—"people are dying." Importantly, this is not because of clinician error but because health care programs and systems have not put proven methods in place, leaving clinicians to manage care on their own. The Henry Ford Health System, Centerstone, and the Institute for Family Health have demonstrated reductions from baseline suicide rates of 60 to 80 percent. Hogan also made the point that Zero Suicide is a package made up of elements, each of which is known to be effective. "It makes sense that the overall package would work, because the elements work if they're done with fidelity." The Zero Suicide model includes an organizational assessment that is also a fidelity tool, Hogan said. A New York study of about 200 clinics found that clinics with higher fidelity scores had fewer suicides. This makes sense, he said, but we need more data to shift the late adopters.

The website zerosuicide.com lays out the basic tools needed to advance. In addition, leadership and elbow grease are critical, Hogan said. "The really big problem is getting health care to say it's our responsibility to keep our patients alive" from this form of preventable death. Behavioral health settings are "starting to get up the adoption curve," but primary care, emergency departments, and health care systems are "just at the beginning."

Suicide risk is linked to but is distinct from other mental disorders, Hogan concluded. Interventions aimed at depression or bipolar disorder are important but not sufficient. Well-established interventions for suicide care now exist, and integrated treatment that attends to both mental illness and suicidality is likely to be more effective. Successful programs like Zero Suicide provide a care pathway and a protocol for treating and managing suicide risk that are embedded within clinics. These interventions need to be integrated "into the work of every mental health practitioner" and into health systems and settings, Hogan stated.

INTERNATIONAL ACTIONS ON SUICIDE PREVENTION

How does a movement spread, how does it produce action, how does it inspire people, asked David Covington, chief executive officer and president of Recovery Innovations, Inc. One way is through international declarations.

In 1989 a small group of people with diabetes, policy makers, and physicians gathered in a rural Italian village and conceived of an audacious proposal: that diabetes management should consist of co-management between an individual and a physician. "This vision has largely been realized," said Covington. Many people no longer remember "when you had to go to a physician to get a blood level." Today people with diabetes are, as expressed in that 1989 statement, co-responsible for their treatment.

In 2002, a small group gathered in the United Kingdom and decided to follow the model of the diabetes pioneers. They proclaimed that an individual having a first episode of psychosis would quickly move from diagnosis to treatment to recovery and live an ordinary life. Though the United States is still making progress on early intervention programs, the time to treatment after a first episode of psychosis in the United Kingdom has been slashed to a target of 22 days, "in large part because of an audacious vision and a pathway for beginning to make that happen."

The 2011 report *Suicide Care in Systems Framework* (Clinical Care and Intervention Task Force and National Action Alliance for Suicide Prevention, 2011) could have gathered dust on a shelf, said Covington. But people involved in the production of the report were inspired by the declarations emerging from international summits. In 2015, representatives of 13 countries produced the document "Zero Suicide: International Declaration for Better Healthcare," which has been viewed many thousands of times throughout the world.[1] At the same time, a series of global zero suicide summits began in 2014 in England, and the summits have grown in size

---

[1] The declaration is available at http://riinternational.com/wp-content/uploads/2016/03/zerosuicidedeclaration_2015draft.pdf (accessed November 27, 2018).

and scope ever since. Subsequent summits have been held in Atlanta (2015), Sydney (2017), and Rotterdam (2018), and the next summit is scheduled for the United Kingdom in 2020.

About the time of the first summit, peer leader Eduardo Vega said at a meeting Covington attended: "I don't know that I am so much against suicide. But here is what I am definitely against: people dying alone and in despair." This statement has become a platform for work going on around the world. In addition to the website zerosuicide.com mentioned by Hogan, the website zerosuicide.org is simultaneously creating a hub for innovation, Covington observed. It brings together not just the people normally involved in suicide prevention but educators, designers, and innovators who can help create an international dialogue and move the process forward.

Today, 90 organizations are part of the Zero Suicide Alliance in the United Kingdom, forming a confederation of providers who can exchange information and guidance. A current challenge is to take the movement into middle- and low-income countries and especially into Africa and South America.

FUNDING ISSUES

In response to a question about securing adequate funding for such initiatives, Hogan pointed out that the Substance Abuse and Mental Health Services Administration's (SAMHSA's) suicide prevention grants now provide more funding than has been the case previously. Also, a small but important part of the 21st Century Cures Act was an adult suicide prevention program authorized for funding of $10 million per year. "This is a starting point," said Hogan.

In addition, much of the progress to be made depends on redesigning the care that now exists, he explained. The suicide prevention activities that need to be done are not complicated, he added, but they have previously been out of scope and health care professionals, including behavioral health professionals, have not received training on them.

Finally, ways need to be found to get reimbursement for these activities, Hogan said. Currently, providers need to figure out setting by setting how to bill for suicide prevention activities. How do they bill for the development of a safety plan? How do they bill for follow-up?

Covington discussed the initial fear among some of the leaders of health care organizations that more screening and assessment would identify more individuals at risk, which would lead to a reduction of profitability. However, he and others had a hypothesis that the opposite would occur: that when health care professionals do not feel confident in their skills they unnecessarily push people in directions that result in increased and avoidable psychiatric inpatient hospitalization. The zero suicide approach can produce a significant reduction in more intensive services for those most in need, he said. Furthermore, the savings may be ever greater at a system level.

Coffey responded by saying that more funding to address this problem cannot be expected. Therefore, "we're going to have to fix it ourselves, we're going to have to find the dividend in the work that we're doing currently." Stopping things that do not work will provide savings that can be invested in things that do work. He also mentioned the "heretical" idea that more screening is not necessarily the answer. "Screening has a place," he said, but providers can spend "way too much time worrying about screening and the precise [risk] number. . . . Instead cut back on that and devote the resources to safety planning and getting much better at means restriction."

RESISTANCE TO THE IDEA OF A ZERO SUICIDE GOAL

Nadine Kaslow, professor of psychiatry and behavioral sciences at the Emory University School of Medicine, asked about the unanticipated consequences of zero suicide initiatives. Could they be a setup for failure and lead critics to question the overall initiative? On a related note, does the identification of people at risk of suicide in hospitals, with the constraints it puts on their autonomy and their identification as high risk, lead to humiliation and stigmatization, she asked.

Hogan responded that "I'm getting pretty old, I don't have that much time, which leads me to say I don't have time for [resistance]. I'm only interested in who wants to do something and what do you want to do now." The other panelists had similar responses. Covington drew a distinction between half measures and full measures. For 70 years the Golden Gate Bridge did some things that saved lives, but it remained a very unsafe place. Finally, after many deaths and considerable pressure, the operators of the bridge decided to install nets extending from the sides of the bridge to stop people from using it for suicide. "They decided in their backyard they were going to take full ownership and do everything they could do. That's what we're really talking about for health care for which we're responsible."

E. Coffey responded that the zero suicide movement needs skeptics and that it is okay to be skeptical about zero suicide from a scientific perspective. But dealing with these criticisms takes time, and "as leaders we have to make a distinction between whether what we're hearing is healthy skepticism versus cynicism." This cynicism is not conducive to building a culture where people are asked to swing for a home run every time they come up to bat. "We have to build a safe environment where people are encouraged to innovate and be bold and audacious, but also at the same time to learn from mistakes."

On the issue of stigmatization, Hogan lamented the sterile environments in hospitals that can result from suicide prevention efforts, such as eliminating ligatures that might be used in suicide attempts. But "morally, we can't not eliminate that." Health care systems also need to replace the things missing because of suicide prevention with other things that will be supportive and relationship centered, he said. Covington pointed out that the company for which he is chief executive officer runs 50 crisis programs and wellness programs in about 5 states, and these programs look different as a result of people with lived experiences being a substantial part of the staff. The people who are in the programs are referred to as guests rather than patients. "It's more like a retreat than it is an institution, more like a home."

Many people, including health care providers, have a fear of suicide and try to distance themselves from patients who are at risk, Hogan said. The presence of this fear suggests two fundamental tasks, he added. One is to create a culture that seeks perfection but does not cast blame. "That's hard leadership work, but it's foundational." The second thing is to include people with lived experience in the planning, design, oversight, and conduct of this work:

> We all felt that we were changing and learning something as we listened to Taryn. She's not the only person who is a genius about this. A lot of people who have been through this experience have that to contribute.

ACTING ON THE EVIDENCE

Richard McKeon of SAMHSA said that a central part of the Zero Suicide initiative has been its recognition of the accumulating evidence that focusing only on an underlying mental health condition is insufficient to prevent suicide among those with such conditions. Suicide prevention needs to be a specific focus, he maintained. At the same time, behavioral health treatment within the health care system takes place in many contexts other than zero suicide programs, and these other contexts may have implications for preventing suicide among those with serious mental illness. "Should we be looking for ways to insert suicide prevention into those initiatives that are going to continue with or without suicide prevention?" he asked. "Is there a way that standard care for depression in primary care could be made more suicide mindful, or early intervention for psychosis?"

E. Coffey responded that one way to embed such care across the health care system is to focus on the safety plan:

> I don't think safety planning should be limited to people who are patients in the mental health care system. I would argue that every patient needs

a safety plan. Aren't those with cancer at risk for suicide? I would start there. If you were to do one thing today that would make a difference in suicide care, I'd take becoming very serious about safety planning for every patient in our health care system.

Hogan responded with an anecdote about a Zero Suicide training boot camp, which they call Zero Suicide academies. One of the people attending the training was an internist in a small practice who seemingly would not need to know this level of detail about suicide prevention. When Hogan asked him at the end of the day what he thought, the internist responded, "Well, I don't deal with this every day, but here's what I'm thinking. The risk of this looks a lot like the risk for my patients of prostate cancer. There's not a lot of that, but where there is, it's pretty important." He said that he was planning to add the suicide question to his Patient Health Questionnaire. Most of the time the responses will be negative. "But if there's a concern, my staff will bring it to my attention, and I'll make that the main focus of what I do with that patient in that visit." Hogan thought that this was a brilliant response. "This is the big lift in primary care."

With regard to specialty care, Hogan responded that the evidence demonstrates that anyone with a diagnosed mental disorder or receiving a behavioral treatment should be asked about suicide. If this generates a concern, actions need to be taken. "That's a big change in primary care in emergency department settings, but we think that's what the evidence today suggests."

Finally, the moderator of the panel, Justin Coffey, vice president and chief information officer at the Menninger Clinic, commented on the safety provisions that have been installed at the Golden Gate Bridge. The netting installed beneath the bridge is not just about aesthetics.

> It's about what the net says, and what the net says is that we have a serious problem in this country. People don't want to have to be reminded of that when they look at the netting, but it's a reminder that we have a serious cultural problem, and it's on one of our most significant engineering achievements. It's such a contrast that people can't accept it, and that's at the heart of their problem.

The Zero Suicide effort has a similar issue. E. Coffey said:

> Part of my worry personally about zero suicide is that when you talk about diabetes and about heart disease, those are natural consequences of health conditions and aging. They can be seen and framed within the natural process. When we start to talk about suicide and mental health, people don't see it the same way. It's about culture and the impact of our culture, and I'm concerned about our willingness to accept those things.

REFERENCES

Ahmedani, B. K., M. J. Coffey, and C. E. Coffey. 2013. Collecting mortality data to drive real-time improvement in suicide prevention. *American Journal of Managed Care* 19(11):e386-e390.

Clinical Care and Intervention Task Force and National Action Alliance for Suicide Prevention. 2011. *Suicide care in systems framework*. Washington, DC: National Action Alliance for Suicide Prevention.

Coffey, C. E. 2003. Pursuing perfect care in neuropsychiatry: Implications of the Institute of Medicine's "Quality Chasm" report for neuropsychiatry. *Journal of Neuropsychiatry and Clinical Neurosciences* 15:403-406.

Coffey, C. E. 2006. Pursuing perfect depression care. *Psychiatric Services* 57:1524-1526.

Coffey, C. E. 2007. Building a system of perfect depression care in behavioral health. *Joint Commission Journal of Quality and Patient Safety* 33:193-199.

Coffey, M. J., and C. E. Coffey. 2016. How we dramatically reduced suicide. *NEJM Catalyst*. https://catalyst.nejm.org/dramatically-reduced-suicide (accessed December 6, 2018).

Coffey, C. E., M. J. Coffey, and B. K. Ahmedani. 2013. An update on perfect depression care. *Psychiatric Services* 64(4):396.

Coffey, M. J., C. E. Coffey, and B. K. Ahmedani. 2015. Suicide in a health maintenance organization population. *JAMA Psychiatry* 72:294-296.

Denchev, P., J. L. Pearson, M. H. Allen, C. A. Claassen, G. W. Currier, D. F. Zatzick, and M. Schoenbaum. 2018. Modeling the cost-effectiveness of interventions to reduce suicide risk among hospital emergency department patients. *Psychiatric Services* 69(1):23-31.

Hampton, T. 2010. Depression care effort brings dramatic drop in large HMO population's suicide rate. *JAMA* 303(19):1903-1905.

IOM (Institute of Medicine). 2001. *Crossing the quality chasm: A new health system for the 21st century*. Washington, DC: National Academy Press.

Klonsky, E. D., B. Y. Saffer, and C. J. Bryan. 2018. Ideation-to-action theories of suicide: A conceptual and empirical update. *Current Opinion in Psychology* 22:38-43.

Millner, A. J., M. D. Lee, and M. K. Nock. 2017. Describing and measuring the pathway to suicide attempts: A preliminary study. *Suicide and Life-Threatening Behavior* 47(3):353-369.

Simon, G. E., C. M. Rutter, D. Peterson, M. Oliver, U. Whiteside, B. Operskalski, and E. J. Ludman. 2013. Does response on the PHQ-9 Depression Questionnaire predict subsequent suicide attempt or suicide death? *Psychiatric Services* 64(12):1195-1202.

Stanley, B., G. K. Brown, L. A. Brenner, H. C. Galfalvy, G. W. Currier, K. L. Knox, S. R. Chaudhury, A. L. Bush, and K. L. Green. 2018. Comparison of the safety planning intervention with follow-up vs usual care of suicidal patients treated in the emergency department. *JAMA Psychiatry* 75(9):894-900.

Van Orden, K. A., T. K. Witte, K. C. Cukrowicz, S. R. Braithwaite, E. A. Selby, and T. E. Joiner. 2010. The interpersonal theory of suicide. *Psychological Review* 117(2):575-600.

Williams, S. C., S. P. Schmaltz, G. M. Castro, and D. W. Baker. 2018. Incidence and method of suicide in hospitals in the United States. *Joint Commission Journal on Quality and Patient Safety* 44(11):643-650.

4

Military Service Members and Veterans

> **Points Made by the Presenters**
>
> - As with the general population, the suicide rate for active duty service members and veterans has increased in recent decades, despite the emergence of effective interventions. (Colston)
> - Seamless transitions between settings and spaces are essential, especially transitions between clinical and community-based care. (Colston)
> - The Department of Veterans Affairs is moving beyond a hospital-based model to a comprehensive public health approach to help meet the needs of the overall veteran population. (Franklin)
> - Within this effort, selective and indicated interventions include expansion of mental health care services and eligibility, lethal means safety training, expansion and dissemination of the Veterans Crisis Line, and enhancement of discharge planning and follow-up. (Franklin)
>
> NOTE: These points were made by the individual workshop presenters identified above. They are not intended to reflect a consensus among workshop participants.

The third and fourth panels of the workshop looked at two specific populations at high risk for suicide: military service members and veterans (summarized in this chapter) and Native Americans and American Indians (summarized in Chapter 5). Examining the issues surrounding these populations reveals both how different populations have different challenges and how some interventions can be effective across all populations.

PREVALENCE AND INTERVENTIONS

Suicide rates have been going up for veterans as well as for the general population, said Mike Colston, captain in the U.S. Navy Medical Corps and director of Mental Health Programs in the Health Services and Policy Oversight Office of the Department of Defense (DoD). As noted in Chapter 2, among states reporting in the National Violent Death Reporting System, every state, except for Nevada, had an increase in suicide rates between 1999 and 2016, with increases ranging from 6 percent to 58 percent (Stone et al., 2018). In the 27 states where veteran suicide rates could be ascertained, 17.8 percent of those who died by suicide were veterans. When Colston was an intern at Walter Reed Medical Center in 1999, the suicide rate within DoD was about 10 per 100,000. Eighteen years later, the suicide rate in DoD had roughly doubled, and the rates among reservists and Air and Army National Guards were even higher. "Suicide is the number one killer of active duty service members right now," Colston said. "It is a huge public health problem and one that we have, despite a lot of resources and real passion, failed to get on top of."

DoD and the Department of Veterans Affairs (VA) oversee populations that are predominantly male, Colston acknowledged. But in 1999, even with an 85 percent male population, the DoD suicide rate was lower than in the civilian population. Since then, the demographics have remained fairly constant, yet the increase in suicide "has been discouraging, to say the least." A rare encouraging sign is that the rate has not changed in 6 years, after a precipitous increase in the late 2000s. "We're stable, but we're stable and high."

Based on clinical experience and the existing evidence, Colston pointed to the effectiveness of cognitive behavioral therapy, dialectical behavior therapy, and other cognitive and problem-solving therapies in some groups, including in people who have engaged in self-directed violence. He also cited the effectiveness of some medications, including lithium, clozapine, and ketamine (see the previous chapter). Caring communication after hospitalization or emergency department contact is inexpensive, sensible, and buttressed by research involving home visits and follow-up contacts, he said.

Suicide is a low base rate event, is often superseded by other clinical conditions, and does not always need to be the focus of clinical concern,

Colston pointed out. He described several patients he has seen during his career who presented as being suicidal and depressed but were in fact delirious because of underlying medical problems. In this regard, he noted that the use of a single instrument can distort clinical priorities. He described his experiences with a young girl who had the prodrome of a borderline personality style and had an "alarming" score on the Columbia Suicide Severity Rating Scale. Colston said that he thought she should undergo dialectical behavior therapy at another facility, but instead she was committed to a hospital where she could learn about other ways to engage in suicidal acts. "Whenever we think of a screening instrument, especially an instrument that's used in isolation, we need to bring those clinical concerns to our clinical prioritization."

Provider monitoring is evolving with technological advancements, and care and monitoring protocols could be generalized across settings, he said. For example, prescription monitoring programs at the state level are powerful tools. "We need to bring some of that capacity for provider monitoring into across-the-board treatment."

Opportunity costs need to be assessed with any rollout, he observed, especially in primary care clinics and emergency departments. An emphasis on suicide prevention can have benefits in such settings, "but what I worry about is where the resources are going." Could other conditions be missed?

Seamless transitions between settings and spaces are essential, he said. In addition, many people not just in clinical care but in mental health care feel that their treatments are stigmatizing and that they want to get confidential care. Or perhaps they want care from a chaplain or from the community, said Colston. "We need to find a way to make sure that we get warm handoffs between not only the clinical space but back and forth between community spaces and clinical spaces." One way to do that is to turn everyone from a member of a universal population to a member of a selected population, such as by offering everyone in a school a cognitive behavioral therapy program.

DoD does not do much screening, but it does do a lot of outcome measures, according to Colston. Without good evidence on the usefulness of screening, this focus on outcomes is "a sensible thing," he said. For example, a focus on outcomes in a behavioral health data portal allows outcome measures to be validated and subsequent care to be standardized and optimized.

DoD offers care, including psychiatrists, psychologists, and social workers, in operational units and in primary care clinics. Colston also called attention to a recent randomized controlled trial showing that enhanced treatment as usual (E-TAU) was equivalent to Collaborative Assessment and Management of Suicide (CAMS) in a suicide cohort. "I have a sense we're doing some of the right things," Colston said.

Colston cited the study by Lubin et al. (2010) that showed a decrease in suicide rates after a policy change that reduced access to firearms in adolescents in the Israeli Defense Forces. The study functioned as a randomized controlled study with equivalent intervention and control groups. "In essence, they took the weapons away from the kids on weekends. The suicide rate stayed the same during the weekdays, and it went down on the weekends. It was a powerful message about controlling access to guns." The intervention, however, was delivered in an optimized setting, which limits its generalizability. In addition, Israel does not have easy access to weapons in its civilian population and weapon owners are trained to safely store and use their weapons. The United States, in contrast, is "awash in weapons," and even though the DoD population is prescreened for mental health conditions prior to entry, the availability of guns offsets that advantage. "Of course, there are constitutional protections around weapons ownership and a number of bigger political issues that come up again and again."

The vast majority of this problem must be addressed in a universal setting, Colston concluded. The list of community stakeholders in a military setting is wide, and this is a community-based problem. DoD does have the means to succeed in community-based interventions. For example, its opiate overdose death rate is one-quarter of the civilian rate, and its rate of opiate use disorder rate is probably one-tenth of the civilian rate. "The solution is leadership," said Colston, "so we have zero tolerance around use." In addition, the military has a focus on pain control, has good law enforcement, and has a force with "a smaller suite of civil rights than your civilian population does."

Even as research proceeds both within the military and outside it, program evaluations and reviews of the evidence base are essential, said Colston, and strategy revisions should stem from these efforts. "We need to look at programs that aren't working, and we need to create a 'stop doing' list, because clearly we're doing a number of things in suicide prevention right now that aren't working."

"First do no harm," Colston said. Though the evidence base is thin for postvention, it *can* do harm, he insisted, if people talk about the means of death or memorialize the setting in which a person died. "Those are things that we really need to look at."

Colston suggested emphasizing the biggest moving parts with resources and efforts, including access to weapons, and then moving on to the 1 percent group. From a systems viewpoint, it is difficult to manage 80 separate problems simultaneously, he said.

A PUBLIC HEALTH STRATEGY TO REDUCE SUICIDE AMONG VETERANS

Keita Franklin, national director of suicide prevention for the Office of Mental Health and Suicide Prevention in the VA, put the prevalence of suicide among veterans in a somewhat different context. Of the 123 Americans who die on average each day by suicide, 20 are veterans, including 1 to 2 active duty service members. Of these 20 veterans, 6 have been receiving care from the Veterans Health Administration (VHA) before their death by suicide, and 14 have not. (Overall, roughly half of veterans receive health care through the VHA and half do not.) Besides improving on the 6 veterans per day who die by suicide despite the best efforts of the VHA, "we have to work outside our system," said Franklin. "Our charge is to prevent veterans' suicide among the whole 20 million population."

Franklin listed several characteristics of veteran populations at increased risk:

- Over age 50
- Women
- Survivors of military sexual trauma
- In a period of transition
- With serious or chronic health conditions
- With exposure to suicide
- With access to lethal means

Of these populations, she noted, the largest in size is veterans over age 50, but the highest suicide rates are among 18- to 34-year-olds. She also called attention to veterans who are in periods of transition, including the period right after leaving the military. To reduce the difficulties of this period, the military has made progress with a transitional program to prepare veterans for career readiness. "They know how to dress for success and they know how to interview properly," she said. But "questions remain about whether or not they know how to adjust to the social aspects of no longer wearing the uniform. . . . Periods of transition are rocky." DoD research has been studying the first year after leaving the military, and this research is now being extended to years 2 through 5, with the initial results being prepared for release at the time of the workshop.

Franklin listed these risk factors for suicide:

- Prior suicide attempt
- Mental health issues
- Substance abuse
- Access to lethal means

- Sense of burdensomeness
- Recent loss
- Legal or financial challenges
- Relationship issues

Franklin also listed protective factors for suicide:

- Access to mental health care
- Sense of connectedness
- Problem-solving skills
- Sense of spirituality
- Mission or purpose
- Physical health
- Social and emotional well-being

To minimize the risk factors and boost the protective factors, the VA is moving beyond a hospital-based model to a comprehensive public health approach. As Franklin described, it has developed a very broad public health strategy to reduce suicide, drawing on a wide range of social science. It incorporates health, psychology, sociology, criminal justice, spirituality, and business (see Figure 4-1). "We're trying to draw public health activities and actions that are measurable and build a more robust evidence base for broad public health strategies," Franklin said.

As part of this strategy, it has adopted universal, selective, and indicated prevention efforts. For example, its universal interventions include the establishment of critical partnerships, public service announcements, and social media campaigns. Its selective interventions include a mental health hiring initiative, lethal means safety training, mental health care for other than honorably discharged veterans, an executive order to expand veteran eligibility for mental health care, "telemental" health, and Veterans Crisis Line information printed on VA canteen receipts. Its indicated interventions include discharge planning and follow-up enhancements, expansion of the Veterans Crisis Line, and postvention follow-up care for family members and friends of someone who has died by suicide.

An important question for a health care provider to ask is "Are you a veteran?" Franklin observed. That question can open the door to someone getting into the right care channels. Franklin said:

> There's no wrong door for care. I don't want you to think the takeaway is that we're trying to singularly identify those at risk and bring them into our system alone, because we're not. We're thinking, if they're at risk, we want them to get care where they want to get care, and of course the best care possible.

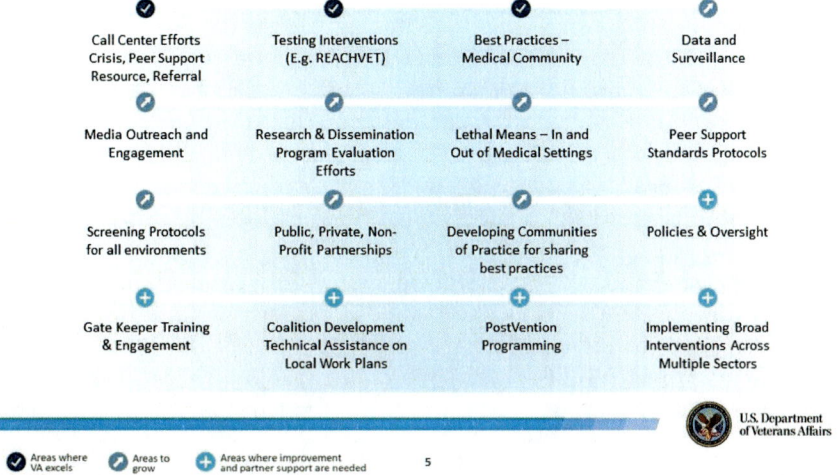

FIGURE 4-1 The Department of Veterans Affairs is pursuing a comprehensive program of suicide prevention.
NOTE: REACHVET = Recovery Engagement and Coordination for Health–Veterans Enhanced Treatment.
SOURCE: Presented by Keita Franklin on September 11, 2018, at the Workshop on Improving Care to Prevent Suicide Among People with Serious Mental Illness.

A recent study found that those in VA care do better than their counterparts in non-VA care (Price et al., 2018). "But if we can get them into some sort of system of care that's good in quality and meets the standards of all things you would expect for your own family member for care, that's what's important."

Franklin discussed in more detail the Recovery Engagement and Coordination for Health–Veterans Enhanced Treatment (REACH VET) program, which uses data to identify veterans at high risk of suicide, notifies VHA providers of the risk assessment, and allows providers to reevaluate and enhance veterans' care. Those engaged in REACH VET have more health care appointments, fewer inpatient mental health admissions, and lower all-cause mortality, she said.

The VA has recently published a *National Strategy for Preventing Veteran Suicide 2018–2028*,[1] which notes that clinical and community-based programs and providers have a critical role to play by screening veteran patients for mental illnesses and alcohol misuse, routinely assessing vet-

---

[1] The strategy is available at https://www.mentalhealth.va.gov/suicide_prevention/strategy.asp (accessed November 27, 2018).

eran patients' access to lethal means, getting educated on military culture and veteran-specific issues and risks, linking veterans in crisis with appropriate services and support, and communicating and collaborating across multiple levels of care. It is not the VA's strategy but a national strategy for preventing veterans' suicide, she emphasized. It calls for "meeting veterans where they live and thrive. We will come to you and, and we will bring capabilities to bear for you."

The VA also provides a spectrum of forward-looking outpatient, residential, and inpatient mental health services across the country. The *VA Office of Mental Health and Suicide Prevention Guidebook* highlights information on these services and related programs that address the mental health needs of veterans and their families.[2] In addition, the VA has a community provider toolkit with free online training for veterans issues, including military culture, for health care providers.[3] It has a suicide risk management consultative program that provides free consultation for any provider who serves veterans at risk for suicide.[4] In collaboration with PsychArmor, the VA has prepared a 25-minute basic training that people can take online.[5]

The Veterans Crisis Line and the Military Crisis Line have been expanding and have been getting about 2,000 calls per day, with 60 to 70 saves being made each day, said Franklin. "They're doing extraordinary work. They're also trying to leverage peer support in doing that and thinking through the way ahead in this space." One effort, for example, has been to have veterans post risks online.

FACTORS SPECIFIC TO MILITARY SERVICE MEMBERS AND VETERANS

In response to a question from Allison Barlow, director of the Johns Hopkins Center for American Indian Health, about why suicide rates are going up, Franklin said that half of the people in active duty who end their life by suicide have a diagnosed mental health or substance abuse problem, but half do not, though behavioral health autopsies find other stressors, such as relationship, financial, or workplace problems. Roughly the same split appears to occur among veterans, she said, though the stressors may

---

[2] The guidebook is available at https://www.mentalhealth.va.gov/about/guidebook.asp (accessed November 27, 2018).
[3] The toolkit is available at https://www.mentalhealth.va.gov/communityproviders (accessed November 27, 2018).
[4] The program is available at https://www.mirecc.va.gov/visn19/consult (accessed November 27, 2018).
[5] The video is available at psycharmor.org/courses/s-a-v-e (accessed November 27, 2018).

be different in an older population. That is why interventions need to be "both and," she said, since the risk factors for suicide are varied.

She also noted that of the 20 who die by suicide, 1 to 2 are active duty but between 3 and 4 are nonfederally activated National Guard, such as firefighters or emergency responders. Colston elaborated on this by noting that the Guard population includes people who have had military training and know how to use weapons. They have a higher suicide rate than active duty or reserved personnel, "so I'm very concerned about that population and how we reach out to them and get them services." Many members of the National Guard have more tenuous economic lives, he noted, "they're struggling as they move from job to job and among activations." They have a smaller suite of social supports than regular Army members. But the secular trend in suicide is still not well understood, he noted, much less the trend within the military. Contagion appears to be playing a part, "but we don't have a good enough understanding."

He added that stigma is still "a huge issue and one that we haven't done well enough on." For example, the fear that soldiers will lose their security clearances because of a mental health diagnosis is prevalent, though this happens very rarely.

In response to a question about whether the attributes of military personnel or veterans have changed over time—for example, after 9/11—Colston noted that the Defense Manpower Data Center collects extensive demographic data, and the trend has been toward military personnel who are more educated and have fewer problems than in the past. The population is still 85 percent male and 15 percent female, as it was in 1999. Integrating females into more roles would reduce the suicide rate in the military, he noted, because the rate is lower in females than in males. He also noted that people wanting to join the military can get waivers for many medical conditions, including mental conditions, and that people who have waivers do just as well as those who do not have them. The more important issue, he thought, is to separate out people in initial training who probably will not do well in the military, which he noted is less common than it used to be. "We used to separate 4,000 people a year for personality disorders; we now separate 300 a year, so the sense is we can retain and treat, [though] I don't know that we're doing all that well on that."

PROVIDER TRAINING, NEEDED SERVICES, AND ACCESS TO CARE

In response to a question on training providers to provide effective care for people with suicidality, Franklin observed that surveys have shown that roughly 60 percent of people across multiple health care professions reported that they were not prepared to engage with suicidality. Given that suicide has a low base rate, they should not be expected to use these skills frequently, but they need to have the skills when necessary, said Franklin. Training needs to be "appropriately resourced" so it is not "one and done."

She also cited the need to engage veterans' family members as gatekeepers. If they know the signs and symptoms of suicidality, they can help get someone into care. "We've not done enough on that side of it."

Colston cited the need for community-based services in addition to clinical services. Of course, comorbid mental health conditions need to be treated, because, as he said, "as a clinician I never see someone who is suicidal who doesn't have a comorbid mental health condition." But suicide can occur in the absence of such a condition, as with adjustment disorders in adolescents that can lead to sudden decisions. At the same time, he warned, both clinical and community-based services need to be evidence based to ensure they are effective.

In response to a follow-up question about how to reach veterans who are not receiving care through the VHA, Franklin advocated a "whole of government" and "whole of industry" approach. "We have to leverage the nation around this problem." A good example is the mayor's challenge work going on with the Substance Abuse and Mental Health Services Administration (SAMHSA), which has brought together the VA and SAMHSA in eight cities to take broad public health approaches with careful evaluations to track outcomes over time. Such studies can reveal whether the best approach is using public health to get people into a clinical environment or whether broad support for public health will make a difference in and of itself. For example, some people may only be willing to go to their church for support. "Might that be okay as the end solution, or is it up to the church to then get them into a clinical setting?" Colston picked up on that point, observing that chaplains have to know how to render mental health care. He also reiterated the value of the crisis lines, which are a good way to reach people who are not getting medical care. The effects of such interventions need to be studied much more carefully, he acknowledged, saying:

> We can't live without those. Those lines are giving care right now to people who either think that the care that they get is too stigmatizing or who we can't match well with someone who can help them.

Michael Schoenbaum, senior advisor for mental health services, epidemiology, and economics in the Division of Services and Intervention Research at the National Institute of Mental Health, asked about the logistical and policy issues associated with identifying veterans who are not receiving care from the VHA and transferring them into the VHA system, to which Andrew Sperling, director of legislative advocacy for the

National Alliance on Mental Illness, added a question about veterans who have received a less than honorable discharge. Both Franklin and Colston noted that checking whether someone who claims to be a veteran actually is a veteran and qualifies for benefits is difficult to do in health care institutions, though a new VA policy is seeking to facilitate this identification. The VHA also offers crisis stabilization for those who have less than honorable discharges. This group is particularly at risk, noted Franklin, yet few come to the VHA system for help. "We have more work to do on marketing and outreach to make sure people know that they're able to come in," she said. "If people have left under other than honorable, they can get care at no cost and we'll stabilize them and help them."

REFERENCES

Lubin, G., N. Werbeloff, D. Halperin, M. Shmushkevitch, M. Weiser, and H. Y. Knobler. 2010. Decrease in suicide rates after a change of policy reducing access to firearms in adolescents: A naturalistic epidemiological study. *Suicide and Life-Threatening Behavior* 40(5):421-424.

Price, R. A., E. M. Sloss, M. Cefalu, and C. M. Farmer. 2018. Comparing quality of care in Veterans Affairs and non-Veterans Affairs settings. *Journal of General Internal Medicine* 33(10):1631-1638.

Stone, D. M., T. R. Simon, K. A. Fowler, S. R. Kegler, K. Yuan, K. M. Holland, A. Z. Ivey-Stephenson, and A. E. Crosby. 2018. Vital signs: Trends in state suicide rates—United States, 1999-2016 and circumstances contributing to suicide—27 States, 2015. *Morbidity and Mortality Weekly Report* 67(22):617-624.

5

Native Americans and Alaska Natives

> **Points Made by the Presenters**
> - Native communities have high levels of unmet mental health needs, with rates of mental illness higher than the general population and a critical shortage of qualified providers. (Barlow)
> - Substance abuse overlaps extensively with Native deaths by suicide. (Barlow)
> - Effective suicide prevention is culturally tailored to the population it serves. (Allen)
> - Comprehensive suicide prevention approaches, with universal, selected, and indicated components alongside robust surveillance and a strong mandate for reporting, can contribute to substantial reduction in suicide rates. (Barlow)
> - In a health care system example, the Southcentral Foundation of Alaska uses integrated primary care teams, case management, telemedicine, local community and behavioral health aides, specialty behavioral health services, and programs specific to suicide prevention, all supported by a strong data collection and analysis process and an independent research team. (Shaw)
> - Interventions need to be targeted at all levels of human experience, respect autonomy, and honor community, which requires that they be tailored to or developed from within local cultures and patterns of being, communication, and relationship. (Shaw)

- In another health care system example, when the Native American Community Clinic in Minnesota identifies those with mental health needs and suicidal ideation, they make available behavioral health providers, spiritual care, and care coordinators who are part of the community. (Myhra)
- Meeting mental health needs requires workforce development, including the training of behavioral health providers, community health workers, and people who can provide peer support. (Myhra)
- Protective factors in these communities, which often get lost in discussions that focus on risk factors, can potentially offer solutions for both suicide risk and serious mental illness. (Shaw)

NOTE: These points were made by the individual workshop presenters identified above. They are not intended to reflect a consensus among workshop participants.

Another population discussed in detail at the workshop was Native Americans and Alaska Natives. As with veterans, these groups have many distinctive attributes, but experiences with effective suicide prevention programs in these groups also bear lessons that apply to all groups.

UNMET NEEDS AMONG NATIVE AMERICANS AND ALASKA NATIVES

Much can be learned from Native American and Alaska Native communities about how to prevent suicide, said Allison Barlow, director of the Johns Hopkins Center for American Indian Health, despite some of the complications that surround the study of these groups. Rates of suicide are much higher among American Indians and Alaska Natives compared with other populations in the United States, but these groups also exhibit great regional differences in mental health and suicide. American Indians and Alaska Natives typically have poor access to mental health services, and epidemiological data on serious mental illness are very incomplete for these groups. In addition, Native groups have cultural differences in understanding mental illness and mental health promotion, which contribute to differences in patterns of suicide. All these factors point to the need for tailored strategies of suicide prevention among Native Americans, said Barlow.

The Indian Health Service (IHS) is responsible for providing essential medical and mental health services for approximately 2 million American Indians and Alaska Natives who are eligible for these services. At least 3 to 4 million other American Indians and Alaska Natives living in urban areas are not covered by the IHS, though they might be covered by Medicare or Medicaid. Historical traumas, including forced relocations and cultural assimilation, broken treaties, and other social, economic, and political injustices have helped to create large behavioral and mental health disparities for American Indian and Alaska Native communities, Barlow observed.

As with other groups, the suicide rate among American Indians and Alaska Natives has been increasing since 2003. In 2015, their suicide rates in 18 states participating in the National Violent Death Reporting System were 21.5 per 100,000, more than 3.5 times higher than those among the racial or ethnic groups with the lowest rates. Suicide is the second leading cause of death behind unintentional injuries for Indian youth ages 15 to 24 residing in IHS service areas and is more than three times higher than among the general population. "The years of productive life loss for those communities is astounding," said Barlow. Natives experience serious psychological problems more than the general population, with the most significant mental health concerns being high prevalences of anxiety, depression, substance use, and posttraumatic stress disorder (PTSD). Though effects of historical trauma on serious mental illness are unknown, American Indians and Alaska Natives experience PTSD at twice the rate of the general population. Men have high alcohol dependence rates compared with other populations, and women have higher depression rates. Furthermore, many of these mental health needs remain unmet, with at least seven times the level of unmet needs in some Native populations for certain illnesses compared with the general population. As a specific example, Barlow pointed to a study of parents revealing much higher rates of serious mental illness among American Indians and Alaska Natives (Stambaugh et al., 2017). "When you think about historical trauma compounded by intergenerational transmission of serious mental illness, we have a huge problem in tribal communities."

Finally, these communities have a critical shortage of qualified treatment providers, especially for children and adolescents, said Barlow. Some regions have no psychiatrists, psychologists, or social workers taking care of tribal community members. In other regions, providers often become overwhelmed by the continuous demand for services, resulting in large vacancy rates. "This gives you some background" of the problems facing Native communities, Barlow said.

CULTURALLY TAILORED INTERVENTIONS IN ALASKA NATIVE COMMUNITIES

Universal prevention efforts need to be part of the mix of an effective response to the public health crisis of suicide in Native communities, said James Allen, professor in the Department of Family Medicine and

Biobehavioral Health at the University of Minnesota Medical School, Duluth campus. Suicide is different among Native communities compared with other racial and ethnic groups. It peaks in adolescence and young adulthood and falls thereafter, rather than staying stable or rising over time (see Figure 5-1).

Suicide in Native communities "calls for a different approach," said Allen. "That's why culture matters."

Allen does most of his work in Alaska, where age-adjusted suicide rates are about 40 per 100,000 people, versus about 18 for Alaska non-Native populations statewide and 14 for the white population across the United States. Suicide is also much more common among Native males, who have a suicide rate that exceeds 60 per 100,000 people in the state. However, Native culture in Alaska exhibits great geographic, language, economic, environmental, and historical diversity, and the suicide rate varies as well by region and within regions. "Suicide is not a problem of Alaska Native people," Allen observed. "It's a problem for some Alaska Native people."

Alaska Natives also share many social determinants of health, including marginalization, intergenerational trauma, and rapid involuntary change, along with culturally distinctive protective factors. Some communities have not had a death by suicide for 30 years, while others have seen waves of

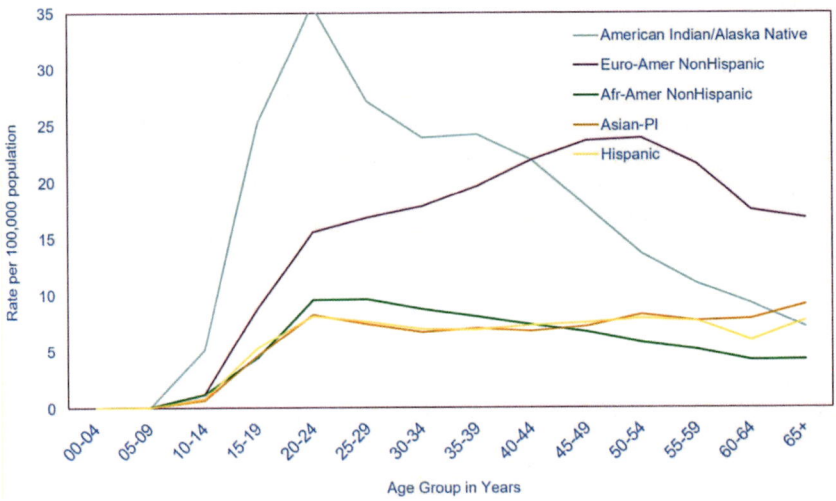

FIGURE 5-1 The suicide rate for American Indians and Alaska Natives peaks in adolescence and young adulthood.
NOTE: Afr-Amer = African American; Euro-Amer = European American; PI = Pacific Islander.
SOURCES: Presented by James Allen on September 11, 2018, at the Workshop on Improving Care to Prevent Suicide Among People with Serious Mental Illness. Data provided by Alexander Cross, Centers for Disease Control and Prevention, 2014, used with permission.

suicide. This emphasizes the need to think about the communities and populations at risk, Allen said.

Allen and his colleagues have been working in Yup'ik communities in Alaska to develop an Alaska Native toolbox designed for local community adaptation. Known as *Oungasvik*, the toolbox makes use of a traditional model of social organization known as *Qasgiq* that seeks to grow protective factors contributing to reasons for life and sobriety (Allen and Mohatt, 2014; Allen et al., 2018). Allen showed a video at the workshop that outlined the basic features of the *Qasgiq* model, which he said is "built around the concept of how do you bring a community together again."[1] It is not a risk reduction approach; rather, it promotes protective factors in young people through a multilevel intervention in families, communities, and individuals.

As an example, Allen briefly described an implementation strategy for a community-level change process. In traditional Yup'ik culture, the *Qasgiq* was a house where all the men lived that provided a central place for community gatherings, ceremonies, and celebrations. Today, the *Qasgiq* model provides a framework for bringing people together with traditional teachings and values to address contemporary challenges. The idea is that "I can solve my problems by seeking out others in my social environment to assist me in solving them," Allen said. By emphasizing community, the model "becomes very culturally patterned and grounded in local cultural beliefs." Research has demonstrated that the targeted protective factors function as predictors of the intervention's two ultimate variables: reasons for life, and reflective processes about the consequences of alcohol consumption or reasons for sobriety (Allen et al., 2014). Community-level factors are the strongest predictors of outcomes, and higher levels of interventions exhibit higher levels of protection.

Effective suicide prevention is culturally tailored to the population it serves, Allen concluded. Culture provides protective factors as tools for prevention, and cultural practices provide effective implementation strategies.

SUICIDE PREVENTION IN THE WHITE MOUNTAIN APACHE TRIBE

The White Mountain Apache tribal community includes about 17,000 tribal members in central-eastern Arizona. They are geographically isolated, have a spectrum of traditional and mainstream cultures, and are governed by an 11-member tribal council that has just selected its first chairwoman. The community has had a 38-year relationship with the Johns Hopkins

---

[1] The video can be viewed at http://www.nationalacademies.org/hmd/Activities/MentalHealth/SuicidePreventionMentalIllness/2018-Sep-11/Videos/Panel-4-Videos/20-Allen-Video.aspx (accessed November 27, 2018).

Center for American Indian Health focused on infectious disease, behavioral and mental health, and training programs. Barlow described some of the work the center and the tribe has done on suicide prevention, especially as it relates to tribal-specific data and tribal sovereignty.

As in other Native American and Alaska Native populations, suicide rates prior to 1950 were very low and then started to rise, with spikes in youth suicide in the late 1980s that have continued until the present. The community has a variety of strengths that it has brought to bear on this problem. It has tribal sovereignty, which provides a degree of autonomy over legislation related to tribal governance. Families are the center of culture, and large family networks strengthen the community. Traditions support the sacredness of life and youth, and the community has a strong capacity to adopt, adapt, and diffuse innovations.

In response to the rise of suicide, in 2001 the tribe mandated a suicide surveillance and registry system. The first registry was a paper-and-pencil reporting system with limited follow-up and financial resources. In 2004, the tribe asked the Center for American Indian Health to help develop a computerized registry management system that could make quarterly reports and help plan responses to ongoing trends. The system has evolved greatly since then, said Barlow, and today all community members, including schools, departments, and individuals, are responsible for reporting individuals at risk for any self-injurious behaviors.

Reportable behaviors include suicide death, suicide attempt, suicide ideation, nonsuicidal self-injury, and binge substance use. These behaviors are followed up on by a team called Celebrating Life. They make a referral, based on the preferences of those individuals, to local services, which can range from local behavioral mental health services to traditional healers to churches. The local case managers started as paraprofessionals and have continued their professional development, with two now enrolled in a Ph.D. program at Arizona State University, so "It is a ladder for development," said Barlow.

The surveillance data showed an average suicide incidence rate of 40 per 100,000 people per year, which is comparable to the rate in Alaska. However, among young people ages 15 to 24, the rate was 130 per 100,000 people, or 13 times the U.S. average. The highest death rates were for 20- to 24-year-olds, and the highest attempt rates were for 15- to 19-year-olds. Males accounted for six times as many deaths by suicide as females, but their attempt rates were similar, which is different from the patterns in the general U.S. population, noted Barlow, where females attempt suicide at three times the rate of males.

To gain a deeper understanding of the precipitants of suicide attempts, Apache research staff conducted a one-time, in-depth, quantitative assessment battery of 71 youth ages 10 to 19 who recently attempted suicide, with a subsample participating in year-long qualitative interviews. "We didn't find anything really incredible or remarkable," reported Barlow. The subset of youth who participated in the diagnostic interview reported higher levels of separation anxiety, agoraphobia, conduct disorder, alcohol dependence, and marijuana dependence. When asked about their reasons for attempting suicide, 35 percent cited family problems, 19 percent said they were angry or depressed, 16 percent said they had relationship problems, 15 percent said they had a recent suicide or death of another person, and 22 percent simply said "nothing," which occurred most often when someone woke up from an alcohol or drug use binge and could not remember having attempted.

Of the youth who attempted suicide, 64 percent were referred to local behavioral health systems, but only 60 percent of those attended. "That means that less than 40 percent of the total who attempted ever got any medical health care," noted Barlow.

Suicide and substance abuse overlap extensively in Native deaths by suicide. Of those who died at ages 10 to 25, 68 percent were drunk or high at the time, and the percentage could be much higher, since the alcohol and drug use of the others was largely unknown. Of those who attempted suicide, 44 percent were drunk or high, and that was not their primary method. Many of the suicide deaths in this community are by hanging, Barlow observed, which implies that means restriction is not a good public health solution in this community. Impulsivity and reactivity were common among those who attempted suicide: "It just happened out of nowhere." "I didn't really think about it, I just took off and tried to look for that rope." Family dynamics and substance use were other frequent themes: "Our relationship is a boat, and it's got holes in it." "I always stayed with my grandma. I only wanted to be around my mom when I knew she was trying to quit. And it wasn't that long before she would take off and drink more."

Since 2001 the tribe has expanded the mandate for reporting, which has shaped its prevention methods, Barlow said. The resulting Celebrating Life prevention program has universal, selected, and indicated components. The universal component includes community-wide education to promote protective factors and reduce risks. The selected component includes early identification and triage of high-risk youth. The indicated component includes intensive prevention interventions with youth who attempt suicide and their families.

As more detailed examples, Barlow listed the following activities under the program's universal component:

- Interagency meetings
- A public education multimedia campaign
- Suicide prevention walks

- Suicide prevention conferences
- Door-to-door campaigns
- Booths at health and tribal fairs
- Regular distribution of lifeline cards

Selected and indicated activities include caretaker trainings, cultural and strength-based activities led by elders, a middle school curriculum taught monthly by elders, elementary school workshops, and field trips. Two brief interventions of 2 to 4 hours are designed to reduce imminent risk and connect to care with a video and curriculum entitled "New Hope"; these interventions now also target substance abuse.

These interventions have had a major effect. From 40 per 100,000 people in the period of 2001–2006, the suicide death rate among the White Mountain Apache Tribe dropped to 24.7 during the period 2007–2012, a 38 percent drop (Cwik et al., 2016). "Comprehensive prevention approaches appear to be helping and working," said Barlow. But serious concerns remain. For example, young women, especially young mothers, seem to be at increasing risk. "This is a huge worry for the tribe." Continuing to build on the strengths of the community will be the key to further progress, she concluded.

SUICIDE PREVENTION IN SOUTHCENTRAL ALASKA

Alaska has the highest rate of suicide in the nation, noted Jennifer Shaw, a senior researcher at Southcentral Foundation. Suicide is the 10th leading cause of death nationally, but it was the fifth leading cause of death in Alaska in 2015. Between 2000 and 2009, of 281 communities in Alaska, at least 1 suicide occurred in 179. With a population of just 740,000 people—17 percent of whom are Alaska Natives or American Indians—there were 200 deaths by suicide in the state in 2015, and 32 percent of those deaths were among Alaska Natives and American Indians.

Reducing the incidence of suicide is among the family wellness corporate initiatives of the Southcentral Foundation, which is one of 12 regional Native corporations and health centers in Alaska. An Alaska Native–owned and Native–operated health care system serving 65,000 people in the greater Anchorage area and 55 rural villages, the Southcentral Foundation covers a region of 107,000 square miles, from the Canadian border to Anchorage to portions of the Aleutian Islands. The vision of the Southcentral Foundation, which recently won its second Baldrige Award and hosted the Surgeon General at its primary care center, is "a Native community that enjoys physical, mental, emotional, and spiritual wellness," and its mission is to "work together with the Native community to achieve wellness through health and related services." The people other systems would call "patients" it calls customer-owners who have a shared responsibility for health and wellness.

The Southcentral Foundation emphasizes integrated care teams in which a primary care provider works alongside a nurse case manager, certified medical assistant, dietitian, and behavioral health consultant with colocated psychiatry and pharmacy services. Behavioral health care services comprise about 13 specialty programs, including outpatient services, residential treatment for substance use issues, treatment for adults with serious mental illness, intensive case management, and behavioral health aides. The system is supported by a strong data collection and analysis process, and it has an independent research team that is largely federally funded.

The Southcentral Foundation has taken a number of steps to address the suicide crisis within the communities it serves. It has established a behavioral urgent response team (see "Overcoming Barriers to Treatment" in Chapter 6), has integrated behavioral health into primary care, has organized a depression collaborative, has instituted a suicide prevention plan, and has signed a memorandum of understanding with the state of Alaska to share suicide data. In addition, specific services are focused on suicide prevention, including the Quyana Clubhouse, which integrates primary care with behavioral interventions, colocated and integrated care in shelters for adolescents and adults, a specialized suicide prevention intensive case management program called Denaa Yeets', traditional healing, and complementary medicine.

The Southcentral Foundation uses telemedicine heavily to provide services to its 55 rural communities, Shaw noted. Telemedicine also lends itself to the caring contacts approach, which focuses on making people stronger and more connected and can be delivered cheaply over distances. "It doesn't require people to travel hundreds and hundreds of miles when they're in crisis," she said. "We can prevent that by providing care when they're at home." Telemedicine also is an important part of workforce development, because it allows providers such as community health aides, behavioral health aides, and dental health aides to stay in their home communities.

The research done by the Southcentral Foundation on suicide prevention is largely clinical and focused on the population it sees in the health care system. It is testing a culturally tailored version of caring contacts with three other tribal sites in the lower 48 states, with the Alaska site being the largest in the study. It was planning to apply a predictive algorithm developed by the Mental Health Research Network to determine whether the algorithm can be validated with a smaller population or whether a population-specific algorithm is needed. The foundation also is thinking about the ethics as well as the logistics of applying such an algorithm, which is a "question that we need to start addressing as a community of researchers and practitioners."

Shaw listed a number of challenges the system faces, including early detection and identification of individuals in need of care; the availability of resources (as she pointed out, "jail is not suicide prevention"); integration between electronic health records, care coordination, and dual diagnosis; continuous coordinated engagement of high-risk individuals; the lack of culturally appropriate, acceptable, and owned interventions; and insufficient funding and scientific support for building a culturally driven evidence base.

She concluded by describing some of the lessons emerging from the foundation's work in Alaska. One is that "trust must come before treatment. Whether you're doing community-based work or clinical work, the relationship is the basis for any healing process or intervention or prevention that's going to happen," particularly with communities that have experienced historical trauma, mistreatment, and maltreatment by researchers as well as clinicians. Communities need to be engaged as partners, teachers, and researchers, she said, while also working on capacity building. In the research department in which Shaw works, 70 percent of the staff are Alaska Native or American Indian, and two of the Native master's-level researchers recently started Ph.D. programs while one was headed to medical school. "Although I'm not a Native researcher, I hope that someday I can put myself out of a job."

Finally, interventions need to be targeted at all levels of human experience, respect autonomy, and honor community, she said, which requires they be tailored to or developed from within local cultures and patterns of being, communication, and relationships.

SUICIDE PREVENTION IN MINNESOTA

"The community that I am working in is ground zero for the opioid epidemic in Minnesota," said Laurelle Myhra, director of behavioral health at the Native American Community Clinic (NACC), who discussed suicide prevention efforts among the Red Lake Nation in Northern Minnesota. Minnesota Natives are five times more likely to die from a drug overdose than their white counterparts, disparities that are linked to the intergenerational effects of historical trauma and cultural genocide and a lack of access to Native providers and culturally specific trauma-informed care. In the past, grandmothers or other family members might have stepped up when a parent was struggling with alcohol use. "What we are seeing now, with the opioid epidemic, is that families are using together," said Myhra.

When someone comes to the clinic, whether for dental, medical, or behavioral health, the clinic screens for depression, suicidal ideation, anxiety, and other conditions. It then rescreens those with depression and suicidal ideation on a regular basis. A behavioral health provider is available for medical and dental visits "or, if they are not willing, a spiritual care person." The clinic has an elder in residence full time who can provide that service or serve as a care coordinator. The elder in residence has started an elder council that reviews policies and procedures and looks for ways to improve planning and care. Those coming out of emergency services receive monitoring and supportive care, and electronic records are available to coordinate care. "Our care coordinators are seen as part of the community," said Myhra. "They work with people's families for years and have a strong connection. That's a real strength."

The clinic has an outpatient behavioral health program that also serves as a training program to build workforce capacity. A peer support recovery program is embedded within the program, and the clinic is working toward certifying and being able to pay the peers. Safety plans include provisions for opioid overdoses. Even when someone is not identified as having suicidal ideation, multiple overdoses call for both a safety plan and care planning and coordination, said Myhra. The clinic seeks to engage families in support and safety planning, and it connects to community supports and events such as ceremonies.

Through partnerships, the clinic has sought to expand access to culturally sensitive and trauma-informed services. One of the most long-standing of these partnerships, with the White Earth Tribe in Minnesota, has been a medication-assisted treatment (MAT) program that includes a clinic prescriber and wraparound services provided through the clinic. This program has been adopted by the tribe as a recovery model, said Myhra. "When people hear that their family members are getting involved in MAT, they get very excited about that and really want to be supportive. That is something different than I've observed in other communities."

Another partnership involves an intensive outpatient program in an impoverished part of Hennepin County, Minnesota. In response to specific gaps within existing culturally specific programs, the partnership works with families and the community to build on existing strengths, to "develop something for those who are in the margins."

In more distant regions where recruiting providers is difficult, telehealth programs are providing diagnostic assessments to people in shelter programs and children's programs. This partnership allows for billing for supportive services such as spiritual care, which has helped with the program's sustainability. In other cases, billing is a major problem, Myhra said. For example, as a federally qualified health care center, the clinic cannot bill for services provided offsite.

Health equity is a major consideration in all the clinic's programs, said Myhra. In addition, meeting the needs of the community requires workforce development, including the training of behavioral health providers, community health workers, and people who can provide peer support. "If we want these providers to be Native American and from the community, we are going to have to train them ourselves, so that's the effort and model that we are moving toward." Finally, meeting needs requires adequate funding, which means asking whether the existing funding is reaching the people most in need.

WORKFORCE PREPARATION

Following up on Myhra's final point, a question about the linkage between care for serious mental illness and suicide prevention focused on workforce development, and specifically on the preparation of people within particular communities to address these issues.

Shaw emphasized the need to start "early, early, early" in building a workforce, well before young people graduate from high school, "because many of these kids are going to be the first in their family to ever leave their family or their village and go to college." She also cited college programs that can direct young people into health care, such as the Alaska Native Science and Engineering Program at the University of Alaska, which sends some graduates to medical school. "Nontraditional" pathways, which are actually traditional in Alaska, are another route to providing health care services. These should be validated using scientific tools and techniques, Shaw urged, so that a growing evidence base can allow them to be funded. "That's going to be a long uphill battle, but those of us who are non-Native researchers and stakeholders have a big role to play in fighting that battle."

Myhra pointed out that many of the evidence-based protocols used in these communities originate in indigenous knowledge. "We have the knowledge within the community," she said, "but we need structures in place to bill for those."

Allen pointed out that each of the projects discussed by the panel also has a capacity development component. "That's part of the picture," he said. "The solutions are within." Communities have cultural knowledge and a past history of success, and local people have the credibility, the cultural understanding, and the trust of the community. "Beginning with that is crucial to being an effective provider."

Finally, Barlow observed that no community in the United States can afford to wait while its treatment needs pile up. "Right now we have great opportunities for early childhood intervention that are intergenerational," she said. "We know that the risk and protective factors start then when someone is pregnant and the family is forming." The Patient Protection and Affordable Care Act is still supporting home visit interventions. In addition, public health nurses and community health representatives can advance suicide prevention, though legislation has been proposed to eliminate community health representatives, "which would be a tragedy." Federal funding streams are supporting these different levels of the workforce and their integration into mental health systems. "That's the future for all communities."

CASE IDENTIFICATION AND MANAGEMENT

In response to a question about the identification and management of individuals who are at high risk for suicide, Barlow elaborated on the White Mountain Apache home visit program. The intention was to go to homes and schools and "meet the people wherever they are, because it was found that that was very much welcome." When suicide deaths among young people began to rise, the behavioral health department and the Celebrating Life team decided to go door to door, which since then has become an annual event. They provide information about resources such as a suicide hotline. They also say, "if you need me now, I can stay. If you need me in the future, I can come back."

Shaw elaborated on the Denaa Yeets' program for people at high risk of suicide. People enroll in the program and participate in its activities while the program checks on them and on their progress. During a series of in-depth interviews with people who had experienced suicide ideation or attempts, many spoke about the critical role that the Denaa Yeets' program played in keeping them alive.

> By knowing that somebody was going to check in on them, by the connection that it provided to cultural activities, . . . to their heritage, to their people, to their community, to the things that feed their soul, [the program] was really important for people who struggled with severe anxiety, with severe depression, and all the other things that we talk about as proximal risk factors.

Lastly, Myhra observed that her clinic offers care coordination and case management through patient advocates who support people with general resources or resources specific to behavioral health care.

PUTTING A SPOTLIGHT ON PROTECTIVE FACTORS

In a final comment, Shaw noted that, while some Alaska Native and American Indian communities have high rates of alcohol and substance use, they also have high rates of abstinence. This bi-modal distribution of risk and protective factors "often gets lost in these discussions." The same may well apply to serious mental illness, she speculated. If the counterparts to such illnesses could be identified, they likewise could be elevated as protective factors in these communities.

I went to Alaska to study suicide among youth, and I quickly realized that I wasn't going to be able to do that as a non-Native outsider who had no relationship with the communities. But after living there for a few years, I realized that that wasn't what needed to be studied.

The conditions of Alaska Native youth are usually so grim that their high suicide rates can seem unsurprising, she said. But "there must be something really right going on in these communities" to be raising so many children who are not just surviving but thriving. "We need to remember the other side of that coin. We need to be looking for those counter factors, . . . because that's where we're going to find solutions."

REFERENCES

Allen, J., and G. V. Mohatt. 2014. Introduction to ecological description of a community intervention: Building prevention through collaborative field based research. *American Journal of Community Psychology* 54(1-2):83-90.

Allen, J., G. V. Mohatt, C. C. T. Fok, D. Henry, R. Burkett, and the People Awakening Team. 2014. A protective factors model for alcohol abuse and suicide prevention among Alaska Native youth. *American Journal of Community Psychology* 54(1-2):125-139.

Allen, J., S. Rasmus, C. C. T. Fok, D. Henry, and the Qungasvik Team. 2018. Multi-level cultural intervention for the prevention of suicide and alcohol use risk with Alaska Native youth: A non-randomized comparison of treatment intensity. *Prevention Science* 19:174-185.

Cwik, M. F., L. Tingey, A. Maschino, N. Goklish, F. Larzelere-Hinton, J. Walkup, and A. Barlow. 2016. Decreases in suicide deaths and attempts linked to the White Mountain Apache Suicide Surveillance and Prevention System, 2001-2012. *American Journal of Public Health* 106(12):2183-2189.

Stambaugh, L. F., V. Forman-Hoffman, J. Williams, M. R. Pemberton, H. Ringeisen, S. L. Hedden, and J. Bose. 2017. Prevalence of serious mental illness among parents in the United States: Results from the National Survey of Drug Use and Health, 2008–2014. *Annals of Epidemiology* 27(3):222-224.

6

Connecting Prevention Along the Continuum of Care

> **Points Made by the Presenters**
>
> - Once someone is identified as having an elevated risk for suicide, the Department of Veterans Affairs (VA) system can call on a variety of effective interventions, but it has difficulty reaching veterans who are outside the mental health system. (Jones)
> - Forms of outreach VA uses include connecting with community organizations and linking the Veterans Crisis Line with local providers. (Jones)
> - The provision of housing can make it possible for people to benefit from the kinds of health care, including behavioral health care, that they need. (Patterson)
> - In doing this work, trust is key. (Patterson)
> - A useful approach is making sure people can control the choices made, such as being involved in developing their own safety plan. (Wocasek)
> - Intensive case management is sometimes essential for people with mental health disorders that have caused them to become disconnected from families and support groups. (Wocasek)
> - Empowering patients to become part of the decision-making process, rather than seeing them as largely passive recipients of care, requires taking the time to develop a relationship with them and pulling in family members, community resources, and other providers. (Wood)

- People with serious mental illness are not well represented in the suicide prevention research and literature, and those in the most complicated circumstances are often explicitly excluded. (Wood)

NOTE: These points were made by the individual workshop presenters identified above. They are not intended to reflect a consensus among workshop participants.

The final two sessions brought the workshop full circle to the role of evidence-based interventions in preventing suicide among people with serious mental illness. In the first of these sessions, four presenters with direct counseling and treatment experience described the approaches they and their organizations take toward individuals with suicidality, including those with serious mental illness. Several of the presenters had their own personal experiences with suicide, which have served as a guide and inspiration for them in developing relationships with their clients.

MULTIPLE INTERVENTIONS IN A DEPARTMENT OF VETERANS AFFAIRS SYSTEM

Nikole Jones, a suicide prevention coordinator with the Department of Veterans Affairs (VA) Maryland Health Care System, was working in a mental health care unit of the VA system in 2006 when a family tragedy changed the focus of her career. She said that she felt "skilled, trained, and confident about assessing for suicide risk," but she did not know that a close family member was struggling in silence. When that family member died by suicide, she decided to become a suicide prevention coordinator, "because I realized that, as a provider-clinician, if I didn't see those signs and symptoms in someone I cared about, I knew it would be impossible for veterans to see it in their peers and for their family members to see it in them."

According to the research, only six veterans who die by suicide per day on average are receiving care through the VA system—of those, only two had received mental health care, Jones pointed out. The system does a good job of assessing veterans at risk of suicide who are receiving mental health care, but it has much less success reaching those outside mental health. Improving suicide screens in primary care and other areas of the hospital can improve identification of risk and access to needed resources, Jones said.

Once someone is identified as having an elevated risk for suicide, the VA system can call on a variety of effective interventions. It makes telephone calls, writes caring letters, and distributes free gun locks for lethal means reduction. The VA system reaches out to churches, community mental health centers, community substance abuse programs, and other organizations to "make sure that the providers working with veterans in the community know the risk that veterans have and the resources that we offer at the VA." The Veterans Crisis Line provides local responders who can determine whether there is imminent risk and, if not, make provider consults.[1] The VA also reaches out to families, such as by letting them know that the Veterans Crisis Line is for family members as well as veterans. "Sometimes the veteran who's at risk may not be willing to get help, or not ready to get help." Outreach workers talk with family members about lethal means restriction, safety planning, and resources that are available.

The VA system has adopted the model #BeThere, which encourages everyone to rally behind our veterans that need support, said Jones. It tries to find out what gives veterans purpose so it can build on their interests and enthusiasm. "For our veterans, we want them to be able to be here tomorrow because their lives are valuable."

BUILDING TRUST THROUGH ADVOCACY AND SERVICES

Alfreda Patterson is a substance use counselor and housing coordinator with Concerted Care Group (CCG) in Baltimore. It is an integrated program, which means "we meet the clients exactly where they are needed." The program provides substance abuse, mental health, psychiatric rehabilitation, and many other kinds of services.

Patterson especially emphasized the group's work on housing, since many of its clients are homeless. The group meets with clients to make sure they are eligible for one of its houses. It also connects them with a variety of support groups organized by CCG, such as groups centered on opioid treatment, mental health, trauma, and grief.

Patterson becomes an advocate for her clients. Whatever they need, she tries to get services for them or send them to other agencies that can meet those needs. CCG also uses a screening tool to identify the services that its clients need and connect them with those services. Again, housing is critical, said Patterson, because once clients are in housing they do much better in treatment. "They go to groups. They are getting jobs." One of her clients was working with the Humane Society; another with a supermarket. "Our clients are engaged."

Patterson said that 22 years ago she was in a situation comparable to those of some of her clients, but "when I needed those services, the services were not available." But through medication-assisted treatment, she

---

[1] The Veterans Crisis Line number is 1-(800)-273-TALK (8255).

was able to go to college, get a degree, and help other people like herself. Patterson said:

> Sometimes [our clients] don't think that I know what I'm talking about, or that a lot of us don't know what we are talking about, because we are book people. But when they find out, "No, I've been exactly where you have been and I feel what you are feeling," they get a sense that "Well, okay, I think I can trust her."

This trust is "the number one key," she said. "You try to get to know them. Therefore, they can get to know you and know that they can depend on you."

OVERCOMING BARRIERS TO TREATMENT

T. J. Wocasek is clinical supervisor for the Southcentral Foundation in Anchorage, Alaska. He oversees the behavioral urgent response team, which is a 24/7 consultant-based team that provides three kinds of services. They address psychiatric emergencies and do risk assessments, for example, of patients who chose not to have a procedure for a life-threatening condition. They are medication providers for patients in the emergency room as well as for outpatients, such as people who have recently been released from the state psychiatric hospital. And they are health consultants who conduct screenings for substance use, depression, grief, and other conditions.

"This is a very meaningful topic to me," said Wocasek. Thirty years ago one of his best friends and teammates died by suicide after school. Adults tried to tell him that it was an accident, but his friend was too smart to work on his car with the garage door down, Wocasek said. "Being truthful is very important, because I got very angry and bitter about the adults trying to protect my feelings rather than just saying what happened." In the next year and a half, before he began college at the University of Arizona, four more of his friends attempted suicide and two died by suicide. "I've been on the other side," he said. He used to think about suicide but asked himself what good he would be if he were dead. "That's why I'm still here, because of that."

He worked as a substance counselor with adults and adolescents and tried to help them get over what he called "thinking errors." When he began working with the Southcentral Foundation, he encountered adolescents who were depressed, impulsive, and suicidal. They would try to avoid their treatment by playing pranks or getting in trouble. "I took that away right away," he said. "I would say, you have two choices. You can either make decisions for your life, or you can have other people make decisions. Other people are judges, police officers, correctional officers, probation officers, doctors, counselors. Which one do you want? I think 100 percent said they want to make their own decisions." That is where treatment begins, he said.

Family values were another barrier to treatment. Coming to Anchorage meant that adolescents would have to adjust to a new culture, where nights are for sleeping and a healthy diet consists of salads and milk, not alcohol and Cheetos. His clients were still loyal to their parents, which created conflict. "I never judged them on that. It was just that here is another way to live your life and live longer." They responded in particular to Native dancing and drumming, which "spoke to them," he said.

Safety planning was emphasized, but Wocasek wanted people to be empowered to develop their own safety plans. He provided them with a template they could use to tell when they were in a crisis, how they could deal with a crisis, and how they would know a crisis is over. As an example of a helpful intervention, he described a system where he has people write on one side of an index card a problem they want to address. Then, on the back side of the card, they write down three to five ways to deal with that problem, whether drawing or listening to music or going for a walk. "You're teaching them how to self-regulate. When they feel in that mood, or that issue comes up, they turn over [the card], they can pick any one, it's their choice, they're empowered to do that, and no one is controlling them."

For some people, intensive case management is essential. Many people with mental health disorders have burned bridges with their families and support groups, so intensive case management is a way to keep an eye on them and not have them go to a hospital to seek help.

TAKING THE TIME TO PERSONALIZE TREATMENT

The day before the workshop, Keith Wood, clinical director of an intensive outpatient service focused on reducing psychotic symptoms through the teaching of positive life-functioning skills, was preparing to leave for the airport when a group of students came to him and said that they were treating a patient who met all the criteria for being suicidal. They needed a licensed clinician to put the person in the hospital. "It has to be quick," he said, "because I have to catch a plane."

The situation he encountered hit at almost every issue discussed at the workshop. With people who have serious mental disorders, a major issue is "do we have time to talk with people like this?" he said. "Do we get paid for doing that, and what is involved? . . . Is suicide really an issue?" The traditional guidance about whether someone may be suicidal does not necessarily fit for people with serious mental illness. Their illness may increase or decrease the likelihood of their being suicidal. If someone with schizophrenia is told that their condition may increase the risk for suicide, they may say, "I don't have schizophrenia. I don't have a disorder." If they accept the fact that they have schizophrenia or some other mental illness, that acceptance may increase the likelihood of their becoming suicidal, Wood said.

The state where Wood works has involuntary commitment procedures, which require filling out forms and getting security involved to put a person in handcuffs and take that person to a hospital. With the patient Wood saw the day before the workshop, other clinicians had joined them in the room, so they could have taken over that process. But, Wood asked, what happens when someone is hospitalized, even if just for a short time? They start losing their power of control. In contrast, the work he does with patients is designed to help them achieve more control over their environment. Thus, making a person a patient could again increase the risk of suicide. "If you take away their power, you take away their hope, you take away their control."

Working with such patients takes time to develop a relationship and express concern, Wood pointed out. It takes time to explain that suicidal thoughts are not abnormal. Much of the work with patients who are thinking about suicide is crisis oriented—how do I protect that person, and how do I protect myself if that person does attempt suicide? "The more we make these individuals feel like they are they and not us, the more we stigmatize them, the more we make them estranged from ourselves, the less we are able to connect with them."

Instead, such patients need to be empowered so they are part of the decision-making process, Wood said. That takes times, and people need to be paid for that time. It requires pulling in family members, community resources, and other providers. It requires developing safety plans and following up with patients to make sure that they adhere to that plan.

Wood did not end up hospitalizing his patient, and he and his colleagues are working with the patient on a safety plan. But this situation exemplified for Wood the challenges of doing prevention with a population that has been seen largely as passive recipients of care. "The way we manage them may have a lot to do with the outcomes that we've been seeing."

GAPS IN AVAILABLE RESEARCH

The moderator of the panel, Andrey Ostrovsky, chief executive officer of CCG, asked the panelists whether enough research has been done on the populations they serve, or whether existing research can be adapted to those populations.

Wood said that he hoped the workshop would cause more research to be directed toward populations like the ones he serves. The people he serves are often explicitly excluded from research—people with multiple diagnoses, people with little education or resources, and people who are homeless. For example, the most dangerous form of suicide involves firearms, but that is not the primary way that people with schizophrenia attempt to take their own lives. People with serious mental illness are "a significant proportion of the people who kill themselves but are not represented in the literature hardly at all." These populations need much more research, he said, such as on ways of infusing prevention into the treatment process.

Jones agreed with that assessment and added that research needs "to talk the same language so we can compare across different groups." For example, younger veterans have different reasons for attempting suicide than do older veterans. Also, predicting who is at risk from suicide is far from perfect. "One person may have a list of risk factors, and it would be too much, and someone else may have a list of protective factors, and it may not be enough." Trying to draw lines around those who are at risk of suicide could miss others who are being drawn to suicide as well, she said.

Wocasek cited a slightly different problem with research on Native populations. Though his colleague Jennifer Shaw (see Chapter 5) conducts research on the work done by the Southcentral Foundation, that research needs to be approved by the institutional review board, and in some cases the board has not approved research involving Alaska Natives because of past abuses involving research.

BILLING FOR SERVICES

Ostrovsky also asked whether any of the panelists had experience with payment mechanisms aligned with the care that needs to be delivered rather than deriving from simple reimbursement codes. Jones responded by saying that the VA is committed to providing suicide prevention care:

> That's our whole role. . . . I'm not going to say, "Well, your hour is up, you have to go, I have someone waiting." They know that we're here for them in that crisis, and I think from their perspective that helps them trust the process and be open about their risk for suicide.

Not rushing the patients and providing enhanced care, as her center does, "makes veterans feel like everyone is working as a team to support them."

Wood responded that he was "jealous of the VA system" and acknowledged that many valuable innovations have emerged from VA systems. "Part of it is because they've been under a more flexible payment system," he said. "There are places in Georgia where we have moved more toward fee for service, which is lethal." If someone is suicidal, the health care system needs to be in contact with that person, said Wood. But a provider calling someone cannot get paid for that call, or a case manager may do something for someone that cannot be reimbursed. Other systems pay for these kinds of activities, and these systems tend to be less institutionalized, less mechanized, and more patient oriented. When systems have more flexibility and people can work more as a team, peers, family members, and other members of a community can be more readily involved in care. "There are systems that do a much better job at that in different points in the country, and we see some of that reflected in suicide rates but also in terms of people adapting to the community and life."

From her perspective as a counselor in CCG, Patterson observed that funding services is less of a factor in her job than in comparable jobs elsewhere. "We have to get paid, but it's all about the clients." If a client needs to be a member of more than one group, the counselors make that happen, regardless of financing. As the chief executive officer of CCG, Ostrovsky contrasted that situation with payment mechanisms in Maryland, which until recently were heavily oriented toward fee for service. If, instead, a lump sum payment could be made for a patient's care, while not the holy grail, providers could work together to do the right thing for people who need care. These alternative mechanisms should be tested, he said, and these tests should be conducted in diverse populations to see how the results of funding mechanisms vary from one group to another.

ONE WISH

Finally, in response to a question about what they would change if they could change just one thing, Wocasek said that enhancing safety and privacy in the psychiatric unit of the emergency room would be his priority. The lack of privacy "is not fair to that patient that other people could potentially be hearing their history and their story." Then he added a second wish: that intensive case management could keep an eye on people in the community and help them get the care they need.

Jones said that she would reduce the stigma surrounding suicide, "and I've been through it personally so I know." When she works at suicide information tables at veterans events, people "see suicide and they just walk on by." If people could talk openly and honestly about suicide, much more progress could be made. One thing she often hears from veterans is that whenever they mention suicide, the automatic response of the health care system is to escort them to the emergency department. If health care providers could respond instead by saying that having the thoughts is one thing and thinking about suicidal behaviors is another, that these thoughts come and go but you can control them, discussions about suicide could be much more open.

Patterson had a similar response, saying that she would like much more transparency in discussions of suicide, both among clients and among providers. "But for them to be transparent, they have to trust me. Every day I say let me see how I can be transparent to them so they can trust me and that way if they trust me I'm able to help them and they're able to receive my help." Finally, Wood said he would shift the emphasis within suicide prevention from pathology to adaptive functioning.

7

Perspectives on the Future Along the Continuum

Points Made by the Presenters

- Partnerships among health care providers, mental health services providers, and community-based self-help groups could increase the availability of suicide prevention services and provide for long-term comprehensive treatment. (Lilly)
- One of the biggest roadblocks to improving suicide prevention is raising awareness that services exist and helping clients understand that they need them, which can sometimes be done better by those who have themselves been directly affected and helped. (Lilly)
- Many resources are now available for health care systems and providers to use that are effective, comprehensive, and directly target people at risk for suicide, but a lack of awareness and training is one of the biggest roadblocks to suicide prevention. (Grumet)
- Health care systems could be better partners in reducing suicide by critically examining and sharing their data on rates of suicide by those for whom they care. (Grumet)
- Investments both upstream and downstream from suicide prevention could link public health and mental health. (Grumet)
- Suicide prevention among people with serious mental illness needs to be in the context of three concentric circles: the professionals who treat people; the institutions that serve people

at risk of suicide who have serious mental illness, including the health care system, the criminal justice system, the child welfare system, and other societal institutions; and the broader community. There are things that can be done in each of these circles. (Evans)

- The implementation of evidence-based treatment, including provider training in suicide prevention for people with serious mental illness, will require substantial investments of resources. (Evans)

NOTE: These points were made by the individual workshop presenters identified above. They are not intended to reflect a consensus among workshop participants.

The final panel was charged with thinking about what could be. It presented three perspectives ranging from the direct patient experience of systems of care and outreach to the design of behavioral health systems at the state and city levels. It included people who represented different facets of the problem and who have crossed multiple boundaries themselves.

OUTREACH AND CONNECTION

Marcus Lilly is an outreach worker for Concerted Care Group (CCG) who educates the community about the services and goals of CCG. These services include a comprehensive approach to substance abuse treatment and mental health services, with the goal of treating a person's entire life and not just a person's addiction. CCG seeks to link potential clients to comprehensive substance abuse treatment and mental health services. As an outreach worker, Lilly deals with people on a day-to-day, person-to-person basis.

In Baltimore, a city that has been called the U.S. heroin capital, Lilly routinely encounters individuals who are on the verge of despair and despondence. Many people in the community suffer from mental illnesses, and suicide is highly associated with substance abuse issues, psychological disorders, and mood disorders, he noted. In addition, drug abuse can often bring about symptoms of mental illness, and mental illness can lead to drug abuse as individuals self-medicate.

One of the biggest roadblocks to improving suicide prevention, he said, is raising awareness that services exist and making clients understand that they need these services. Sometimes his clients laugh at him. "When you're going through withdrawal, you're poor, you're unsafe in your own community, sometimes it's hard to see beyond those issues and realize that you need treatment." People who have been helped can then go on to become advocates for these programs in an "each one teach one" model. "Someone who has been directly impacted by a mental health illness, or a substance abuse issue, or has had suicidal thoughts in the past, is in a better position to reach more people that may be suffering from those same illnesses."

He works from experience, having had suicidal thoughts himself when he was young. "I felt like my life wasn't worth living at one point in time. And, at the same time, I didn't want any treatment. I didn't know I needed treatment, and I didn't have any access to services in my community. I was in my own bubble."

Lilly noted that many people who died by suicide had already reached out to health care providers. Providers therefore need to make suicide prevention a medical priority by providing better awareness and treatment for people who are at risk of suicide, he said. Treatment facilities and medical facilities also could help each other with training, information, and identification.

For many such populations, not many treatment facilities are available. Partnerships between health care providers, mental health services providers, and community-based, self-help groups could increase the availability of suicide prevention services and provide for long-term comprehensive treatment. Also, increased investments in the quality, expansion, and advertisement of these mental health services is needed, he said. Educating church leaders, community leaders, and others in the community about people who are at risk of suicide would help them understand the issues better on a day-to-day basis, including the treatments that are available.

Those at risk of suicide need to believe they have the ability and power to organize and execute plans that would produce positive results in their lives. Creating self-efficacy "is the smallest thing we can do as individuals. Especially as an outreach worker, I try to build on the assets of the people that I encounter."

Lilly also promoted a civic engagement concept that he calls public sociology. This would connect academic universities with everyday citizens to empower members of the community to become co-creators and co-agents of change. Together, researchers, service providers, and community members could "sit around the table and cocreate solutions that will improve suicide prevention." This would help create unity among health care providers, mental health services, and people in the community, he said. It also would empower people in communities to be more proactive in their own treatment processes.

THE DIVERSITY OF AVAILABLE INTERVENTIONS

Julie Goldstein Grumet, director of health and behavioral health initiatives at the Suicide Prevention Resource Center and director of the

Zero Suicide Institute at the Education Development Center, focuses on embedding evidence-based suicide care practices into health care systems. Many resources are now available for health care systems and providers to use that are effective, comprehensive, and directly target people at risk for suicide. But a lack of awareness of these resources is one of the biggest roadblocks to suicide prevention, Grumet said. "Safety planning, screening, treatments like dialectical behavior therapy, cognitive therapy for suicide prevention, follow-up during times of care transitions—despite the fact that the evidence exists to use these, they are vastly underutilized in health care systems." As just one example, she said that she is often astonished that her center does not receive more phone calls from primary care practices. "We know depression is one of the leading issues that people come into their primary care physician to talk about. Yet, frankly, they rarely reach out and say, 'What do you have for me? And please partner with us.'"

Training in suicide prevention is a serious problem, she said. Health care providers are not required to learn about suicide-specific treatment practices in graduate school, and continuing education requirements exist in only a few states. Grumet said:

> Yet, we send our loved ones to get care by providers who we expect are going to be well trained and competent and confident—and the workforce isn't. We have many surveys to attest to the fact that the workforce does not feel comfortable and confident. We don't tolerate that in medical care. We would never send our loved ones to a surgeon who said, "I don't really have any training, but I'm going to try my best." But we do that in behavioral health every day. We send our loved ones to providers who we think are well trained, and they are doing their best, and they absolutely are incredibly caring individuals. But they don't have the skills. They haven't been trained in suicide-specific practices.

Grumet said that she would love to see the Zero Suicide approach adopted throughout health care. "We believe it really is transformative in the health care systems that have adopted it." In the meantime, the National Action Alliance for Suicide Prevention has released recommended standard care practices that health care providers can adopt. National organizations should endorse and distribute these standard care practices, said Grumet, and health care providers should be familiar with them.

Health care systems could be better partners in reducing suicide by critically examining and sharing their data on rates of suicide by those for whom they care. Today, health care systems are not required to share these data, so no benchmarks exist. Such sharing may happen informally, but many systems still do not know how well or poorly they are doing. Making these data publicly available would enable systems to improve.

That has been one of the advances fostered by the Zero Suicide movement, she added—that health care systems are starting to share their outcomes. "But we're at the beginning of that, and we can't take 15 or 20 years to get farther down the road."

Another roadblock is reaching individuals who are not seen in health care. More than half of the people who die by suicide do not have a mental health diagnosis, according to data from the Centers for Disease Control and Prevention. The data also reveal that those who die by suicide, such as middle-aged men, share many characteristics even without a known mental health diagnosis. These shared characteristics provide an opportunity to involve new and nontraditional partners, Grumet said. "We have to be much more creative in thinking about paraprofessionals and peers and other types of community-based efforts."

People also need to be reached in culturally appropriate ways, Grumet said. If they are not going to engage with a health care system, then ways need to be found to reach them where they are more comfortable seeking care.

Despite the challenges, "hope prevails," Grumet observed. With the recent suicide deaths of Anthony Bourdain and Kate Spade, the media ran fewer stories that focused on their traumatic lives or concluded that "they needed to die by suicide." Many more stories focused on where to find help and on how many people have thoughts of suicide but do not go on to kill themselves and live meaningful, quality lives. Grumet said:

> The media is beginning to get it right. This way of communicating about suicide offers hope that those who are at risk for suicide can begin to feel less judged by others, less ashamed, [that they can] come forward with their stories about their suicide experiences or good experiences that they have had.

Such stories help empower the public to know what to do and where to look for help. They break down barriers that can help prevent suicide.

Investments are needed both upstream and downstream from suicide prevention, she observed, which has the effect of linking public health and mental health. Downstream efforts are things like Zero Suicide, the use of robust electronic health records that can capture the work that health care systems are doing, well-trained staff, 24/7 crisis services, and psychiatric emergency rooms, which can reduce the burden on emergency rooms and provide better and more timely care to people with mental health needs. Upstream efforts recognize and address the risk factors that contribute to suicide, including economic despair, lack of connectedness, and exposure to trauma. "We need to work much more closely with the nonprofits, the national organizations, and the organizations that work to address these types of issues," Grumet said. "We work in silos frequently, and we can't expect that things are going to change if we're in silos."

Technology will help. Apps for safety planning or to push out messages of thought and hope and caring for loved ones make a difference. Predictive analytics can target those who might be at greater risk. Social media can lead people to resources and perhaps make it possible to identify people who are at risk of suicide. "There's a whole field still available to us with regard to technology that I imagine will continue to emerge."

Grumet closed with a short-term recommendation and long-term recommendation. The short-term recommendation is that all organizations, from the local level to the state level to the national level, need to know who is dying by suicide and implement interventions to target the highest risk populations. "In the short term, I hope that people will use data and then share their data."

Her long-term recommendation was that organizations collaborate across the different types of challenges in society, whether opioid misuse, domestic violence, or childhood trauma. With the grave public health issues facing Americans today, collaboration will yield faster and greater results.

PREVENTION AT ALL LEVELS

The best way to help people with serious mental illness, said Arthur Evans, chief executive officer of the American Psychological Association and previously the commissioner in Philadelphia for the Department of Behavioral Health and Intellectual Disability Services, is to begin with the entire population. Many people with serious mental illness who are also suicidal are not in position to get help, in part because one of the risk factors for suicide is isolation. If interventions are considered as primarily clinical, without also considering the support services that are needed, "we are missing an opportunity."

The system needs to be aligned with the research, he said, and today it is not. For example, most systems deal with suicidality as a binary issue, but thinking in this way is inadequate. Suicidality exists along a continuum. That is why good transitions are critical, which is a major issue for most systems of care.

Evans often talks about treatment as a black box. "When people have a diagnosis, or need help, they have to come to us, and to our black boxes, to get the help." People are then released back into their communities with little or no help, care, or support. "There are so many problems with that paradigm," Evans said. One of the biggest is that the people who need help often do not come to treatment programs. Therefore, "if all of our efforts are directed at treatment, we are going to miss a lot of people."

Health care systems and service providers need to think outside the box to what is happening to people in their communities, he said. Evans thinks about contexts in terms of three concentric circles. The first includes the professionals, including mental health professionals, who see people who present for treatment and the treatment approaches they use. These people often are not trained to deal with patients who have suicidal thoughts. Nor are many of them trained to deal with substance abuse, which significantly increases the risk of suicide. "There are a whole host of things that we can do in that innermost circle to increase our ability to effectively deal with those people who have suicidal ideation," Evans said. In addition, he pointed out that there is "a big gap between what most treatment programs are doing and what the science says around what works." Substantial investments of resources will be needed to implement evidence-based treatment programs, including provider training. "We are not making the kind of investment that we need if we really want practice change to happen."

The second circle includes the institutions that serve people at risk of suicide who have serious mental illness. Many people with serious mental illness are involved in the criminal justice system, the child welfare system, the health care system, or other societal institutions. Strategies exist to help those systems identify and address mental health issues, but these strategies are not always used. In the criminal justice system, for example, people with serious mental illness are at high risk for suicide. The people in these institutions need training, as do the people in such organizations as churches, synagogues, and mosques. "That's often where these issues start to emerge. Those are the people who are going to provide help and support."

The third circle is the broader community. Clinical care and public health are not mutually exclusive, Evans said. "A good clinical system is the foundation of a good public health approach." At the community level, several things need to be done. One is to reduce the stigma associated with mental health challenges, as other presenters at the workshop noted. "We can build the best treatment programs in the world, have the best outcomes in the world, but if people don't go to them because they are embarrassed, or they are ashamed, or they don't know how to get there, it doesn't matter." This generally requires focusing on things outside health care as well as inside. As an example, he cited community participatory art projects to try to change the narrative—"using storytelling and getting people who have lived the experience to talk about their stories." He has sent outreach workers to community health fairs to perform mental health screenings right next to the person taking blood pressures. "When we first started doing that in Philadelphia, people said, 'People will never come to a table about mental health and start to talk to you.' Turns out that people do. In fact, they are glad we are there." Furthermore, in almost every setting, someone approached the outreach team who was suicidal. "That made me think, what if we were not there?"

THE INFLUENCE OF RESEARCH

In response to a question about the influence of research on his work, Evans said that as an administrator responsible for a system, he relies heavily on research but also understands that people cannot wait for all the research to happen in order to act. For example, evidence exists for what works in particular cultural groups, for people with serious mental illness, and for people demonstrating suicidality. "We have to be able to take all of that and to essentially cook. We have to put things together using our best judgments because we won't always have the studies for the very specific individuals we're working with." In Philadelphia, his department worked with a large immigrant population that did not even have a word for mental health. "We know that there weren't any studies that were done for this population, and we couldn't wait for those studies to be done." At the same time, many things do not translate, and policies are not always implemented effectively. "Even when we know what works, it's really hard to get those things to work in real-world settings."

Grumet addressed the difficulty of maintaining fidelity when small programs are scaled up while maintaining enough flexibility to meet the needs of the targeted population. Fidelity often suffers so greatly that programs are abandoned after a few years and new programs are adopted. Research on how to implement programs with fidelity could help address this problem. "Which part of the recipe can you change, and which part needs to be faithful to the model?"

THE LINK TO INCARCERATION

Lilly, responding to a question about the barriers he faced upon coming out of the criminal justice system, said that he was released from prison less than 1 year before the workshop after being incarcerated for 13 years. "My reentry process was very difficult," he said. His record of being incarcerated and the associated stigma made it hard for him to find a job, housing, educational opportunities, and other resources. What helped him was access to community-based self-help programs as well as to CCG. "That helped connect me to different associations and different institutions within my community, to help support me and help me stay focused on my goals, as well as, of course, being employed. This is a very purposeful feeling." In helping other people, he has been able to help himself. "Helping them talk through their problems, you gain new perspectives on your own problems."

CCG has invested in Marcus to become an advocate on issues that have affected him. Similar investments could help many other people, he said, "with employment, education, vocational training, and a sense of fulfillment. . . . That would help other individuals transition a little more successfully."

Ostrovsky noted that his board was initially opposed to hiring Marcus. They are thoughtful people, he said, but they did not want to have the liability of hiring someone with a history of involvement with the criminal justice system. "They didn't have the benefit of the data of actually interacting with Marcus and going through a rigorous interview process." His hiring has not only brought a valuable skill set into the organization but has contributed to the largest revenue growth in this organization's history. "If Marcus didn't have that background and ability to empathize with our patient population, we wouldn't have had that revenue growth." Employers need to be educated about the immense benefits of hiring people with criminal justice backgrounds, said Ostrovsky. "That's a barrier that needs overcoming."

Evans spoke of a similar experience with health care providers in Philadelphia, where hiring people with lived experience led to greater engagement with patients and greater resources for the program. "The economics worked. To me, that's very strong evidence." The city of Philadelphia ended up creating a toolkit to facilitate the hiring of peers, including people with lived experience.

CHANGING THE COMMUNITY NARRATIVE

In response to a question about changing the community narrative about suicide prevention, Grumet recommended such actions as going into churches and working with other community groups to reach people where they are most comfortable receiving care. This enables reaching out to people even before they have mental health issues. "We want people to feel connected, because then we know . . . if they're struggling, whether financially or workwise or relationship-wise." Community programs also can be replicated rather than invented anew in each community. "Part of the challenge is figuring out the scalability of really effective interventions," said Grumet. She recommended getting stories like Lilly's into national publications and broadcasts so people can hear how peers can make a difference, "because otherwise it feels very challenging for systems to know where to begin. We have many best kept secrets that we don't do a good enough job promoting."

Evans broadened the conversation to include the social determinants of both health and mental health. He noted that most treatment programs do not deal with social supports, even though many studies show that social supports are a strong determinant of health status. "Health care accounts for only 10 percent of our health status," he said, adding:

> The mindset shift that we have to make is to understand what those [other] things are and then use our best judgment around how we can affect those things and collect the data to make sure that what we're doing is actually effective.

He reiterated that one of the biggest challenges for treating people with serious mental illnesses is that they are often isolated and disconnected from people from communities:

> Our experience has been that when we help people to make those kinds of connections, it makes a big difference in their clinical outcomes.... It's not all about symptoms. It's about these broader issues that affect our health.

LINKING SUICIDE PREVENTION TO THE TREATMENT OF MENTAL ILLNESS

Finally, Nadine Kaslow, professor of psychiatry and behavioral sciences at the Emory University School of Medicine, pointed out that the workshop has been about both suicide prevention and serious mental illness. "We need to pull together those worlds much more," she said. Professionals tend to work in siloes that do not interact with each other much. "But people don't live in those silos," said Kaslow. She explained:

> Part of my response to the social determinants is that we need to sit at tables where we're all together to talk about this, because part of that gets to the prevention issue. If childhood maltreatment is one of the biggest risk factors for deaths by suicide in virtually every population and every age and every gender and every race and ethnicity, but we're not doing anything to prevent that, and then we get this downstream issue, there's an issue. We all need to work together on this.

8

Ideas from the Breakout Sessions

At the beginning of the second day of the workshop, the participants broke into two sessions that discussed major topics emerging from the first day's discussions. Participants in one session discussed issues with a focus on what providers need, which also encompassed political leadership. Participants in the other session discussed the financing and other policy issues associated with integrating suicide prevention into care for people with serious mental illness.

CREATING MOMENTUM AT THE STATE LEVEL

Oscar Morgan, project director for the Central East Mental Health Technology Transfer Center, who reported for the first breakout session, noted that many important observations made by individuals participating in the breakout session have been operationalized by the National Action Alliance for Suicide Prevention in its report *Crisis Now: Transforming Services Is Within Our Reach*.[1] Extending these observations, participants in the breakout session discussed the possibility that the Substance Abuse and Mental Health Services Administration (SAMHSA) might send a letter to the governor of each state quantifying the crisis for the nation and for that state. The letter then would suggest implementing the recommendations contained in *Crisis Now* and offer free technical assistance from SAMHSA to do so. SAMHSA's technical assistance centers could develop a uniform

---

[1] The report is available at https://theactionalliance.org/sites/default/files/crisisnow.pdf (accessed November 27, 2018).

implementation strategy that may differ from state to state but that would lead to implementation of a zero suicide approach for people with serious mental illness.

In response to the report from the breakout session, Richard McKeon, chief of the Suicide Prevention Branch in SAMHSA's Center for Mental Health Services, noted that an important issue is the nexus of responsibility between the Centers for Medicare & Medicaid Services (CMS) and the states. "When I talk to colleagues at CMS, one of the things that they emphasize, at least in terms of Medicaid funding, is how much it's a state issue." Clear guidance would be helpful to states, for example, in Medicaid plans. One way to provide this guidance is through strong relationships between mental health commissioners and Medicaid commissioners, he noted. However, he questioned how feasible it would be for SAMHSA to send a letter to all of the governors of the states, though he noted that letters to Medicaid directors have come jointly from SAMHSA and CMS. Perhaps the state secretaries of health and human services would be the most appropriate recipients of such letters, though engaging the nation's governors would also be "critically important."

In this regard, Christine Moutier, chief medical officer of the American Foundation for Suicide Prevention, noted that it has been building a mechanism to encourage all of the states to have a state suicide prevention day in which all the evidence and needed steps could be presented at the state level.

TRANSITIONS IN CARE AND BUNDLED PAYMENTS

The participants in the second breakout session spent much of their time discussing transitions in care—and in particular the transition from an emergency department contact or a psychiatric hospital into the community. Health systems need incentives to focus resources on people with serious mental illness who are at risk for suicides during these transitions, observed Andrey Ostrovsky, chief executive officer of Concerted Care Group, who provided a report from the session. Measuring the factors associated with a good transition raises challenges, he noted. Such a transition involves not just a medical model but consideration of the community, family, and other resources that are involved, along with the provision of adequate support for a good transition.

Participants focused in particular on the use of bundled payments to ensure care continuity across transitions. Precedents exist for such bundled payments, both with public funding mechanisms and with commercial insurance. One challenge noted by several participants is to bring an evidence-based approach to the population of people with severe mental illness who are at risk for suicide. Important factors identified by various participants in the breakout session include appropriate assessment for people at risk of suicide, establishing a safety plan, and making sure that a person has an adequate number of contact points, including family members and community providers.

Participants in the breakout session also discussed ways of providing financial incentives upstream of transitions, such as during contacts with the primary care system or an emergency hotline. As a specific example, could organizations be incentivized to adopt electronic health records in the behavioral health care space, which would facilitate transitions?

Ostrovsky pointed out that bundled payments would be "perfect grounds for an 1115 demonstration" under the Medicaid program. It would have to be done on a state-by-state basis, though the Center for Medicare & Medicaid Innovation (CMMI) could also promote a model that is more comprehensive than Medicaid. He also thought commercial group insurance was a possibility, so long as the financial case can be made either by care savings or by increased market share. If "you get a progressive group or employer-based insurer to take this up, you don't have to wait for a model to be designed by CMMI or through the long process of getting an 1115 demonstration approved."

McKeon agreed that the evidence is solid regarding things that need to be done during the transition period. However, whether this evidence translates to populations other than the ones studied to date remains unknown. For example, does it apply to people with schizophrenia, bipolar disorder, or other serious mental illness? "That's a piece that we don't know as much about."

McKeon added that bundled payments would be "useful and important." In addition, they would provide an opportunity to learn from innovations and move forward. For example, different people have different needs, and some of these needs could be met at little cost, such as text message interventions, while other needs may require face-to-face contact or home visits, "presuming that you have a home."

COMMENTS ON IDEAS FROM THE BREAKOUT SESSIONS

As part of the plenary session following the breakout session, workshop participants commented on several issues raised during the breakout discussions and earlier in the workshop.

Nadine Kaslow, professor of psychiatry and behavioral sciences at the Emory University School of Medicine, pointed to the need to collect data to see how effective different approaches are with people who have serious mental illness and to modify those approaches accordingly. Greater knowledge could bring other funders into the room besides people who fund health care policies, she said.

Amy Loudermilk, state initiatives manager for the Suicide Prevention Resource Center, asked where the responsibility for suicide prevention among those with serious mental illnesses resides organizationally. Is there a need for an organization or formalized collaboration to focus on suicidality and people with serious mental illness, she asked. This population is the responsibility of several different professions but not of a single one.

Jim Allen noted that implementation science has shown the difficulty of getting professionals to buy in, which is crucial to implementing or changing a system of care. He also pointed out that a thoughtful rollout requires local decision making. "There are many models of how you respond to an actively suicidal individual. They all have an evidence base. The important issue is that the provider community in the state pick one so everyone shares the same pathway and shares the same vocabulary. They'll do that if they feel they were part of the decision process in arriving at that." He suggested involving consumers in that decision as well.

Jennifer Shaw, a senior researcher at Southcentral Foundation, reminded the group that people are very diverse and one size does not fit all. While the evidence may be strong in one population, "we need to be very thoughtful about who was included and how it was evaluated for the diverse populations that make up our United States." Research needs to be validated in minority communities (even though they are often majorities) and also be culturally grounded and culturally driven.

Shari Ling, Deputy Chief Medical Officer, CMS, advocated identifying bright spots that are working "no matter where they are." Integrated care offers tremendous opportunities, she said, but people working today have worked out important parts of the answer, and "we can learn from what is working."

Julie Goldstein Grumet, director of health and behavioral health initiatives at the Suicide Prevention Resource Center and director of the Zero Suicide Institute at the Education Development Center, described seeing many best practices and good outcomes occurring on the local level, "but people have a hard time publishing those results and sharing those practices." As a result, these practices and outcomes remain siloed and hidden. One solution would be for journals to reach out and solicit articles about the intersections of people with serious mental illness and suicide. They also could cultivate authors who do not typically submit articles. "We have many state suicide prevention coordinators, tribal elders and leaders, and people in rural areas who have been heroic in finding ways to combat suicides in their communities and have outcomes but have a hard time getting it onto a national stage."

Mike Hogan of Hogan Health Solutions called attention to SAMHSA's new program to provide technical assistance through the National Dissemination Center and the Department of Health and Human Services' region-specific centers. This new technical assistance structure could be extremely helpful because the field is still at an early adoption stage where targeted information is very useful. The evidence base for people with high suicidality is "pretty clear, but it's also new and . . . hasn't been synthesized," Hogan observed. Because suicide is a low base rate event, a randomized controlled trial with suicide as one outcome would be prohibitively large. The existing evidence rests largely on the concept that effective interventions "have achieved bigger reductions in suicide than anything else in the world." Also, suicide prevention programs are made up of components that all have an evidence base.

In addition, Hogan observed that the Interagency Serious Mental Illness Coordinating Committee was considering some of these issues at the same time as the workshop, and it may be a valuable partner in considering these issues. The National Mental Health and Substance Use Policy Laboratory is another innovation-oriented organization that could help drive policy changes.

9

Reflections on the Workshop

At the end of both days of the workshop, individual workshop participants discussed the main messages they heard emerging from the workshop.

THE ELEMENTS OF EFFECTIVE INTERVENTIONS

Research over the past 15 years has demonstrated the need to build on the commonalities of effective interventions, said David Rudd, president of the University of Memphis and member of the workshop planning committee. Mike Hogan identified several of these in his presentation, Rudd noted, including "ask," "engage and act for safety," "reduce lethal means," "treat suicidality," and "provide support when needed" (see Figure 3-4 in Chapter 3). To these, Rudd added compliance facilitation, which is "a part of everything you do." Whenever providers in his institution ask a patient to do something, they have the patient rate on a scale of 1 to 10 how likely they are to do it. If the patient responds with a 1, meaning that the patient is not going to do it, they ask the patient why. "Tell us exactly why you can't do that element of treatment." They then explain why that element is important. "We go back to the model and explain why this is a critical element of treatment and what role it serves."

Another feature of the common elements of effective interventions is they are relatively simple and straightforward, though they may be delivered differently by individuals and organization with different theoretical perspectives. The one modification Rudd suggested is that, as part of safety planning, health care providers teach people how to ask for help. "You can't assume that somebody knows how to ask for help. You have to role play it, you have to walk through scenarios, and you have to help them understand the language of asking for help." Shame "is one of the biggest barriers to compliance," he noted. He and his colleagues elevate that issue and address it with every single person with whom they work.

In addition to the commonalities of effective interventions, Rudd identified three major topics discussed at the workshop: education, clinical delivery, and systems integration. Clear evidence pointing to what should be done exists in each area. The challenge now is not what to do but how to do the right thing organizationally and politically. "We have good foundational places to start; we just need to start implementing." Saying that the problem is complex tells Rudd that someone is ashamed of it, because that means "we'll never solve it, we're not accountable for it, we're not responsible for it, and as a result we don't know what to do." Rudd said that he was encouraged not to have heard a single time at the workshop that the problem is complex.

Rudd observed that the range of material presented at the workshop "demonstrates not only the breath but the creativity of people who are working to meet these challenges—and these are very significant challenges." The task before the field is now to integrate innovative interventions into the care of people struggling with serious mental illness. For example, are innovations more effective within a Zero Suicide initiative or within an integrated wellness effort? Does that help with some of the shame and stigma that prevent people from getting help?

FUNDING AND FOLLOW-UP NEEDS

Andrey Ostrovsky, chief executive officer of Concerted Care Group (CCG), cited the need to fund both research and service delivery. "Suicide prevention, and in particular suicide prevention in people with serious mental illness, is grossly underfunded in order to get the comprehensive approaches that are needed to meaningfully move the needle." One concrete idea emerging from the workshop is bundled payments to help align financing with the desired outcomes. "The more I've been tweeting about it and researching analogs, the more I get optimistic at how doable this will be—especially now [with] the political winds that are blowing." What needs to happen, he said, is to get the people who control policy in the same room with those who oversee the funding of programs to figure out how to implement the science.

Another critical need that he identified is to reduce stigma. The presence of people at the workshop who were willing to talk publicly about their experiences is exciting, he said, because "most people will not talk about [this] publicly, and we have to talk about it publicly. If we don't talk about it publicly, it'll just keep getting stigmatized."

Ostrovsky said that he and CCG are willing to follow-up on the ideas presented at the workshop, whether reaching out to governors or implementing the knowledge that already exists. "We may fail, and that's fine, but let's fail fast, fail cheap, fail often. We have to get out there and do it, not just talk about it, not just publish, but get out there and do it."

COLLABORATION AND TRAINING

Nadine Kaslow, professor of psychiatry and behavioral sciences at the Emory University School of Medicine, wondered why the two main topics discussed at the workshop—suicide prevention and serious mental illness—remain such different worlds when they overlap so extensively. A major way to reduce the distance between them is to create collaborations among stakeholders that represent suicide prevention and the treatment of serious mental illness.

This split is reflected in clinical training, she pointed out. In psychology training, working with people who are suicidal or have a serious mental illness is generally ruled out, while psychiatry training follows the opposite model, giving new trainees responsibility for people with the most serious mental illnesses. Neither of these models "makes a lot of sense to me," said Kaslow. "We need to begin to think in a different way of how do we train people to be prepared to do this work," not just asking them if they are ready to treat people with serious mental illness. One of the reasons Kaslow became interested in suicide was from losing a patient to suicide early in her career, after which she participated in a program run by the American Foundation for Suicide Prevention to meet with others to discuss what happened, including the psychiatry resident with whom she had treated the patient. "It was a pivotal experience for us in terms of healing."

Suicide prevention requires that providers adopt an ecological model encompassing the individual, the family, the clinician, and society, she continued. In that respect, root cause analysis that tries to determine what went wrong "is extremely problematic and difficult." It encourages providers to feel that they have failed and to avoid treating people at high risk of suicide again. An ecological model also emphasizes the importance of culture in treatment, assessment, and prevention, including cultural adaptations to interventions or interventions that emerge from a particular cultural group.

The workshop demonstrated the need to include people with lived experience at the table. In most settings, people still do not feel safe to share their stories, Kaslow said. Creating this safety is critical so meetings do not consist of people who have been identified as having lived experiences and people who have been identified as not having those experiences, since suicidality occurs on a continuum and "we all live on that continuum somewhere."

STAKEHOLDERS, RESEARCH, AND INFRASTRUCTURE

Lisa Jordan argued for the need to include nurses at the table as well, because caring is central to their profession. Some of the first community health workers were nurses, she said, and nurses have constructed models of caring that incorporate patients into the plan of care. In addition, nurses can help other health care providers care for themselves when a patient ends his or her life. "We have to be there with you, because we believe as nurses that we are the conduits to get many of the other professionals that are working with a patient together and to keep everybody abreast."

Scott Dziengelski from the National Association for Behavioral Healthcare called attention to the fact that people with serious mental illness have a much higher mortality rate than the general population. "These individuals are dying 25 years sooner than everybody else in the population," he said. "They've been left out of the longevity revolution. . . . This is part of a greater conversation about serious mental illness and mortality."

James Allen, professor in the Department of Family Medicine and Biobehavioral Health at the University of Minnesota Medical School, mentioned the need to align the Substance Abuse and Mental Health Services Administration's (SAMHSA's) research with that of the National Institutes of Health to study the implementation of the ideas discussed at the workshop. Suicide is a low base rate event, he said, but many distal indicators can be used to identify effective prevention and treatment approaches. Work in fields as distant as process engineering can lead to innovative methods in suicide prevention, he added, which points to the value of collaboration among professions.

Amy Loudermilk, state initiatives manager for the Suicide Prevention Resource Center, emphasized the role of the infrastructure developed by the states for suicide prevention. Working on this infrastructure can elevate the issue and reflect its multidisciplinarity, which Ostrovsky added could be done through such organizations as the National Association of State Medicaid Directors.

COMMITMENTS TO ACTION

Arthur Evans, chief executive officer of the American Psychological Association, like Ostrovsky of CCG previously, committed his organization to following up on the major issues and ideas raised at the workshop. He also observed that the subject matter discussed at the workshop needs to be disseminated as widely as possible so every community has someone who is involved in the issue. Getting people in government, system administrators, and many others involved will be required to influence the social determinants that affect suicide, he said, which will require leadership within many different communities.

In follow-up to the workshop, Christine Moutier of the American Foundation for Suicide Prevention committed her organization to stay engaged in actionable strategies as an outgrowth of the workshop. She reiterated her observations made during the first panel: that the openness and readiness of the nation is ripe, and that health care systems, payers, and policy makers must make the changes needed to meet the public health crisis and the growing demand on the part of patients and families. She observed that the American Foundation for Suicide Prevention is well positioned to advocate for changes like bundled payments for postdischarge care, to cooperatively fund research related to suicide prevention, and to catalyze health systems to implement suicide prevention training and system changes.

OUTCOMES AND TECHNICAL ASSISTANCE

Richard McKeon, chief of the Suicide Prevention Branch in SAMHSA's Center for Mental Health Services, discussed the need to track outcomes. Part of the reason the Department of Defense and the Department of Veterans Affairs have focused on suicide prevention is they have the data about the people they are losing to suicide, and many health care systems do not have those data. In addition, the Interdepartmental Serious Mental Illness Coordinating Committee has recommended generating these data more quickly, he reported, which could further increase accountability. "That information potentially can be made available more quickly than the 2-year wait for the CDC [Centers for Disease Control and Prevention] statistics that specify suicides."

On the data issue, Ostrovsky mentioned a treasure trove of data is available in the form of claims data held by Centers for Medicare & Medicaid Services. These data are available after just 1 month for every state and territory in the nation and could be made available through the Transformed Medicaid Statistical Information System if they were accessed by researchers or other government agencies.

Finally, McKeon cited the new regionally based technical assistance centers being established by SAMHSA as a source of information. The stakeholders in suicide prevention could help guide what the most productive role of these centers would be.

The link between suicide and serious mental illness "will be an abiding concern for SAMHSA over the next number of years," McKeon concluded. "We need to be able to have more of these conversations."

Appendix A

Workshop Agenda

Improving Care to Prevent Suicide Among
People with Serious Mental Illness
The National Academies
2101 Constitution Avenue, NW
Washington, DC

Tuesday, September 11, 2018

8:00 a.m.	**Registration**
8:30 a.m.	**Welcome and Workshop Overview** David Rudd, University of Memphis, *Planning Committee Chair*
8:40 a.m.	**Instructions for Breakout Topic Selection** Bridget B. Kelly, The National Academies of Sciences, Engineering, and Medicine, *Workshop Planning Consultant*
8:45 a.m.	**Opening Session** **Framing Remarks** Richard McKeon, Substance Abuse and Mental Health Services Administration

Why This Matters: A Personal Perspective
Taryn Aiken Hiatt, American Foundation for Suicide Prevention–Utah and Nevada Area

9:20 a.m. **Panel 1: Patterns of Risk and the Prevention Landscape**
Moderated by Andrey Ostrovsky, Concerted Care Group, *Planning Committee Member*

Holly Wilcox, Johns Hopkins University
Christine Moutier, American Foundation for Suicide Prevention

10:30 a.m. **Break**

10:50 a.m. **Panel 2: Suicide Prevention in Health Care Systems**
Moderated by Justin Coffey, The Menninger Clinic, *Planning Committee Member*

Ed Coffey, Baylor College of Medicine
Mike Hogan, Hogan Health Solutions
David Covington, Recovery Innovations, Inc.

12:15 p.m. **Lunch**

1:15 p.m. **Panel 3: Suicide Prevention for Veterans and Service Members**
Moderated by Bridget B. Kelly, The National Academies of Sciences, Engineering, and Medicine, *Workshop Planning Consultant*

Michael Colston, Office of Health Services Policy and Oversight, Department of Defense
Keita Franklin, Office of Mental Health and Suicide Prevention, Department of Veterans Affairs

2:15 p.m. **Panel 4: Suicide Prevention in Tribal Communities**
Moderated by Bridget B. Kelly, The National Academies of Sciences, Engineering, and Medicine, *Workshop Planning Consultant*

APPENDIX A   *105*

                James Allen, University of Minnesota Medical School, Duluth
                Allison Barlow, Johns Hopkins Center for American Indian Health
                Jennifer Shaw, Southcentral Foundation
                Laurelle Myhra, Native American Community Clinic

3:45 p.m.   **Break**

4:00 p.m.   **Panel 5: Connecting Prevention Along the Continuum of Care**
                Moderated by Andrey Ostrovsky, Concerted Care Group, *Planning Committee Member*

                Nikole Jones, Perry Pointe Veterans Affairs
                Alfreda Patterson, Concerted Care Group
                T. J. Wocasek, Southcentral Foundation
                Keith Wood, Emory University, Grady Health System

5:05 p.m.   **Key Messages from Day 1**
                David Rudd, University of Memphis, *Planning Committee Chair*

5:15 p.m.   **Adjourn Day 1**

                Wednesday, September 12, 2018

8:00 a.m.   **Registration and Breakout Topic Sign Ups**

8:30 a.m.   **Welcome and Brief Recap of Day 1**
                David Rudd, University of Memphis, *Planning Committee Chair*

8:40 a.m.   **Instructions for Breakouts**
                Bridget B. Kelly, The National Academies of Sciences, Engineering, and Medicine, *Workshop Planning Consultant*

8:50 a.m.   **Transition to Breakout Rooms**

8:55 a.m.	**Breakout Sessions**
	Facilitated by
	Andrey Ostrovsky, Concerted Care Group, *Planning Committee Member*
	Anne Styka, The National Academies of Sciences, Engineering, and Medicine
	Ashleigh Husbands, Education Development Center
	Bridget B. Kelly, The National Academies of Sciences, Engineering, and Medicine, *Workshop Planning Consultant*
	Jerry Reed, Education Development Center
	Joshua Prasad, Concerted Care Group
	Maia Laing, Office of the Chief Technology Officer, Department of Health and Human Services
	Margeaux Akazawa, Office of the National Coordinator for Health Information Technology, Department of Health and Human Services
	Nadine Kaslow, Emory University School of Medicine, *Planning Committee Member*
10:25 a.m.	**Break and Reconvene in Main Room**
10:45 a.m.	**Breakout Reports**
11:30 a.m.	**Closing Panel: Perspectives on the Future**
	Moderated by Nadine Kaslow, Emory University School of Medicine, *Planning Committee Member*
	Marcus Lilly, Concerted Care Group
	Julie Goldstein Grumet, Suicide Prevention Resource Center
	Arthur Evans, American Psychological Association
12:30 p.m.	**Key Messages from the Workshop Planning Committee**
	Facilitated by David Rudd, University of Memphis, *Planning Committee Chair*
1:00 p.m.	**Adjourn Workshop**

Appendix B

Biographical Sketches

SPEAKERS, PANELISTS, AND FACILITATORS

Margeaux Akazawa, M.P.H., is a program analyst in the Office of Technology at the Department of Health and Human Services (HHS), Office of the National Coordinator for Health Information Technology (ONC). In this role, she is responsible for advancing health information technology strategies and approaches to combat the nation's opioid epidemic. Ms. Akazawa previously worked with ONC's Consumer eHealth and Engagement Division where she led efforts to improve patients' access to their health information through technology. Ms. Akazawa has human-centered design expertise and experience facilitating design thinking trainings including serving as a coach for the HHS Idea Lab Ignite Accelerator program and as a workshop facilitator for the Better Government Movement. Prior to joining ONC, Ms. Akazawa was a Presidential Management Fellow at the Department of Housing and Urban Development where she served as a Desk Officer for Promise Zones, a place-based community revitalization initiative. Ms. Akazawa received her M.P.H. in Behavioral Science and Health Education from Emory University, Rollins School of Public Health, and her B.A. in Anthropology from the University of California, Berkeley.

James Allen, Ph.D., is a professor in the Department of Family Medicine and Biobehavioral Health and senior scientist with the Memory Keepers Medical Discovery Team for American Indian and Rural Health Equity at the University of Minnesota Medical School, Duluth campus. He was previously Associate Director at the Center for Alaska Native Health Research and graduate faculty in the clinical-community psychology program with indigenous and rural emphasis at the University of Alaska Fairbanks, a Fulbright Scholar at the University of Oslo Medical School, and graduate faculty in the clinical psychology program at the University of South Dakota. Research interests include American Indian and Alaska Native community resilience and prevention of youth suicide and substance use risk, community-based participatory research, multi-level intervention, and research methods for small populations. He currently works with Alaska Native communities developing an evidence base for a culturally grounded multi-level intervention promoting protective factors to prevent youth suicide and alcohol risk, and documenting community-level resilience structures promoting youth well-being and protection from suicide.

Allison Barlow, Ph.D., M.P.H., M.A., is the director of the Johns Hopkins Center for American Indian Health. She has worked at the Center since 1991 to co-create and evaluate ecologically sound, evidence-based, and culturally resonant interventions with tribal communities to address behavioral and mental health disparities. Projects to date have spanned the design and demonstration of preventive interventions targeting adolescent suicide, depression, and substance abuse, as well as the design and evaluation of a tribal-specific early childhood home-visiting intervention, Family Spirit, to promote parenting and early child development—with the latest iteration including modules to address early childhood obesity and water insecurity. Other lines of research have included obesity and diabetes prevention, and most recently, youth entrepreneurship to address the twin problems of poverty and poor health trajectories. Her team has succeeded in disseminating successful interventions to more than 120 tribal communities across 19 states. They have also produced pioneering evidence to support the effectiveness of Native community health workers to promote behavioral and mental health, overcome access barriers in low-income communities, and build local human capital through an indigenous workforce.

Ed Coffey, M.D., is a neuropsychiatrist and a professor of Psychiatry and Behavioral Sciences and Neurology at the Baylor College of Medicine, Houston, Texas. Dr. Coffey is an accomplished physician (board certified in both Neurology and Psychiatry) with expertise in neuropsychiatry and brain stimulation, and is consistently listed as a "Top Doctor" by numerous organizations. He is also an award-winning health care executive, recognized for leading high-quality, financially successful, academically based systems of integrated health care. Dr. Coffey's innovative work on "Perfect Depression Care" has been widely cited as a model for health care transformation, and its audacious goal of "zero suicides" has become an international movement, honored by The Joint Commission (2006 Codman

Award), the American Psychiatric Association (2006 Gold Achievement Award), the Malcolm Baldrige National Quality Award (2011), and by his appointment to the National Action Alliance for Suicide Prevention (2011).

Captain Mike Colston, M.D., is the director for Mental Health Programs in the Department of Defense's (DoD's) Health Services Policy and Oversight office. This office seeks to improve the lives of our nation's service members and families through oversight, strategy management, program evaluation, and policy regarding DoD's care of psychological health and substance use disorders, traumatic brain injury, and the clinical management of suicidality. Previously, Captain Colston served as the Director of the Defense Centers of Excellence for Psychological Health and Traumatic Brain Injury. As the director of the Mental Health Program in the Office of the Assistant Secretary of Defense for Health Affairs, Captain Colston oversaw a project that reviewed more than 200,000 cases involving posttraumatic stress disorder and depression diagnoses, led a mental health team in the independent investigation of the Washington Navy Yard tragedy, and co-chaired DoD's Addictive Substances Misuse Advisory Committee. As Chair of the Mental Health Department at Naval Hospital Great Lakes, he oversaw a large-scale clinical integration of the Department of Veterans Affairs and DoD services at the Lovell Federal Health Care Center in the Chicago metro area. During deployment in support of Operation Enduring Freedom, he led a combat and operational stress team that supported a catchment of 10,000 service members. Captain Colston holds a B.S. in Industrial and Management Engineering from Rensselaer Polytechnic Institute and a master's degree in Marine Affairs from the University of Rhode Island. He joined the Navy as a line officer, serving as a nuclear engineer and surface warfare officer aboard USS Carl Vinson (CVN-70), deploying twice to the Arabian Sea and completing a Pacific Rim Exercise. He then commanded a littoral patrol boat as an afloat officer-in-charge. Transitioning to Medical Corps service, he earned an M.D. from the Uniformed Services University of the Health Sciences, trained as a resident in psychiatry at Walter Reed Army Medical Center, and completed a fellowship in child and adolescent psychiatry at Northwestern University. He practices inpatient child and adolescent psychiatry at Fort Belvoir Community Hospital. His military decorations include the Defense Superior Service Medal and Defense Meritorious Service Medal, Surface Warfare and Officer-in-Charge Afloat devices, and campaign ribbons stemming from four overseas movements.

David Covington, LPC, M.B.A., is the CEO and the president of Recovery Innovations, Inc. (d/b/a RI International). He is also a partner in Behavioral Health Link, co-founder of CrisisTech 360 and leads the international initiatives "Zero Suicide," "Crisis Now," and "Peer 2.0." A licensed professional counselor, Mr. Covington received an M.B.A. from Kennesaw State and an M.S. from the University of Memphis. He previously served as vice president at Magellan Health responsible for the executive and clinical operations of the $750 million Arizona contract. He is a member of the HHS Interdepartmental Serious Mental Illness Coordinating Committee established in 2017 in accordance with the 21st Century Cures Act to report to Congress on advances in behavioral health. A recognized health care innovations entrepreneur, global speaker, and blogger, Mr. Covington is a two-time national winner of the Council of State Governments Innovations Award. He also competed as a finalist in Harvard's Innovations in American Government in 2009 for the Georgia Crisis & Access Line, and the program was featured in *Business Week* magazine. Mr. Covington is the President-Elect of the American Association of Suicidology and has served on the National Action Alliance for Suicide Prevention Executive Committee since 2010. He is also the Chair of the National Suicide Prevention Lifeline Substance Abuse and Mental Health Services Administration Steering Committee. He has served on numerous committees and task forces on clinical care and crisis services, including the National Council for Behavioral Health Board of Directors.

Arthur C. Evans, Jr., Ph.D., policy maker, clinical/community psychologist, and health care innovator, is the CEO of the American Psychological Association (APA). Dr. Evans has held faculty appointments at the University of Pennsylvania Perelman School of Medicine and the Yale University School of Medicine. Prior to coming to APA, he served for 12 years as Commissioner of Philadelphia's Department of Behavioral Health and Intellectual disAbility Services where he led a groundbreaking transformation of the Philadelphia service system that significantly improved health care outcomes and saved millions of dollars that the city used to expand services. Dr. Evans has also served in leadership positions in clinical administration and state government in the state of Connecticut where he developed a multidisciplinary private practice.

Keita Franklin, L.C.S.W., Ph.D., a member of the Senior Executive Service, is the National Director of Suicide Prevention for the Department of Veterans Affairs (VA) Office of Mental Health and Suicide Prevention. Dr. Franklin serves as the principal advisor to VA leadership for all matters pertaining to suicide prevention. She leads a team of experts engaged in research, program evaluation, innovation, program development, data and surveillance, and partnerships. Before joining the VA, Dr. Franklin served as the director of the Defense Suicide Prevention Office where she was responsible for policy and oversight of the Department of Defense suicide prevention programs. She is a licensed social worker with a specialization in children and families, and has a Ph.D. in social work with specialized training and certifications from the Center for Advancement of Research Methods and Analysis. Dr. Franklin received a leadership award from Virginia Commonwealth University for leading efforts to help train and advise the social work profession on working with military families.

Julie Goldstein Grumet, Ph.D., is the director of Health and Behavioral Health Initiatives at the Suicide Prevention Resource Center. Dr. Goldstein Grumet provides strategic direction to health care providers to recognize and respond to suicide emergencies. She is also the Director of the Zero Suicide Institute, where she oversees the dissemination, resource development, and application of the Zero Suicide initiative nationally by providing consultation and training to health care systems. Dr. Goldstein Grumet received her Ph.D. from George Washington University.

Taryn Hiatt is a dedicated advocate and shares her story and passion to give hope and educate our communities about suicide. She is a survivor of her own attempts as well as a survivor of suicide loss, losing her father Terry Aiken on October 5, 2002. Ms. Hiatt is a founding member of the Utah Chapter of the American Foundation for Suicide Prevention and currently serves as the Area Director for Utah and Nevada. Ms. Hiatt is a certified safeTALK, CONNECT Postvention and Mental Health First Aid Trainer, facilitating hundreds of seminars to many different groups. Ms. Hiatt is a passionate advocate for change and has been featured in both *U.S. News & World Report* and *The Huffington Post*. She has testified before congressional members in Washington, DC, to increase awareness and support for better access to mental health services and to promote healthy discussions about suicide. She is widely respected throughout Utah for her hard work and dedication to saving lives. Taryn is a recent graduate of Utah Valley University with her Bachelor's Degree in Psychology.

Michael Hogan, Ph.D., served as the New York State Commissioner of Mental Health from 2007 to 2012, and now operates a consulting practice in health and behavioral health care focusing on health care issues with significant public health impact, especially suicide prevention. The New York State Office of Mental Health operated 23 accredited psychiatric hospitals, and oversaw New York's $5 billion public mental health system serving 650,000 individuals annually. Previously Dr. Hogan served as Director of the Ohio Department of Mental Health (1991–2007) and Commissioner of the Connecticut Department of Mental Health from 1987 to 1991. He chaired the President's New Freedom Commission on Mental Health in 2002–2003. He served as the first behavioral health representative on the board of The Joint Commission (2007–2015) and chaired its Standards and Survey Procedures Committee. He has served as a member of the National Action Alliance for Suicide Prevention since it was created in 2010, co-chairing task forces on clinical care and interventions and crisis care. He is a member of the National Institute of Mental Health (NIMH) National Mental Health Advisory Council. Previously, he served on the NIMH Council (1994–1998), as the president of the National Association of State Mental Health Program Directors (2003–2005) and as the board president of National Association of State Mental Health Program Directors' Research Institute (1989–2000). His awards for national leadership include recognition by the National Governor's Association, the National Alliance on Mental Illness, the Campaign for Mental Health Reform, the American College of Mental Health Administration, and the American Psychiatric Association. He is a graduate of Cornell University, and earned an M.S. degree from the State University College in Brockport, New York, and a Ph.D. from Syracuse University.

Ashleigh Husbands, M.A., is a prevention specialist for the Suicide Prevention Resource Center within the Education Development Center. Ms. Husbands provides technical assistance to state and campus youth suicide prevention Substance Abuse and Mental Health Services Administration (SAMHSA) grantees as well as unfunded state suicide prevention coordinators. Ms. Husbands has previously worked as a Regional Suicide Prevention Specialist for the Florida state youth suicide prevention SAMHSA-funded grant, where she provided technical assistance to behavioral health providers on Zero Suicide implementation as well as provided suicide prevention, intervention, and postvention trainings to community members. She also has prior experience as a crisis counselor, answering for the National Suicide Prevention Lifeline. Ms. Husbands earned a master's in clinical psychology from Towson University in 2013.

Nikole S. Jones, L.C.S.W., completed her undergraduate studies in Psychology (minor in Criminal Justice) at James Madison University in 1993 and master's degree in Social Work at Howard University in Washington, DC. She completed her internship at the Department of Veteran Affairs (VA) at the Washington, DC, VA Medical Center. She really enjoyed working with veterans and wanted to commit her career to helping America's warriors. Ms. Jones's experience in the VA includes work in the Substance Abuse Rehabilitation Program (SARP), and as an Inpatient Psych Social Worker. However, after the death of her family member in 2006 to suicide, Ms. Jones became passionate about suicide prevention. During that time suicide prevention became a major initiative in the VA, Ms. Jones accepted a job as the Suicide Prevention Coordinator at the VA Maryland Health Care System. Ms. Jones and the Suicide Prevention Team are committed to providing education to veterans and their families, VA employees, and the local community of the risk, warning signs, and protective factors suicide in an effort to reduce the incidence of suicide and increase access to appropriate care in the VA. Ms. Jones was instrumental in establishment of the Maryland State Chapter of the American Foundation for Suicide Prevention and served as the chapter's first President of the Board of Directors. The Maryland chapter has grown to provide prevention efforts to every county in the state. Ms. Jones is currently working on her first self-help book, *The Compulsion to Die*, that will be available in early 2019. Ms. Jones also has a private practice (Therapy 4 Life) that provides Christian counseling and consultation services.

Maia Laing, M.B.A., is the senior business consultant within the Office of the Chief Technology Officer (CTO) at the Department of Health and Human Services (HHS). In her role, Maia identifies innovative solutions to complex challenges within HHS. Prior to joining the Office of the CTO, Ms. Laing worked for the Centers for Medicare & Medicaid Services on an enterprise effort to implement a process improvement mindset across the center. Ms. Laing holds a deep passion for improving delivery of care and has worked on projects in both federal government and nonprofit settings; including *U.S. News & World Report* top 10 ranked Brigham and Women's Hospital in Boston.

Marcus Lilly is a University of Baltimore college student and an Outreach Worker with Concerted Care Group. As a former incarcerated citizen, he also advocates for prison reform, substance abuse treatment, and mental health services. He is the author of *The Marshall Project's* article, "Finding College by Way of Prison." He has been a guest speaker at the University of Baltimore and Georgetown University. He is the co-creator of "37th and Jessup: Classmates Divided by Bars, United for Justice," which is one of Georgetown University Justice Initiative projects. His goal is to become a mentor and share his story of transformation with high-risk youth.

Richard McKeon, Ph.D., M.P.H., received his Ph.D. in Clinical Psychology from the University of Arizona, and a Master's of Public Health in Health Administration from Columbia University. He has spent most of his career working in community mental health, including 11 years as director of a psychiatric emergency service and 4 years as an associate administrator/clinical director of a hospital-based community mental health center in Newton, New Jersey. In 2001, he was awarded an American Psychological Association Congressional Fellowship and worked for U.S. Senator Paul Wellstone, covering health and mental health policy issues. He spent 5 years on the Board of the American Association of Suicidology as the clinical division director and has also served on the Board of the Division of Clinical Psychology of the American Psychological Association. He is currently the chief for the Suicide Prevention Branch in the Center for Mental Health Services of the Substance Abuse and Mental Health Services Administration, where he oversees all branch suicide prevention activities, including the Garrett Lee Smith State/Tribal Youth Suicide Prevention, Campus Suicide Prevention grant programs, the National Suicide Prevention Lifeline, the Suicide Prevention Resource Center, and the Native Aspirations program. In 2008, he was appointed by the Secretary of Veterans Affairs to the Secretary's Blue Ribbon Work Group on Suicide Prevention. In 2009, he was appointed by the Secretary of Defense to the Department of Defense Task Force on Suicide Prevention in the Military. He served on the National Action Alliance for Suicide Prevention Task Force that revised the National Strategy for Suicide Prevention and participated in the development of the World Health Organization's World Suicide Prevention Report. He is also the co-chair of the Federal Working Group on Suicide Prevention.

Christine Moutier, M.D., chief medical officer of the American Foundation for Suicide Prevention, knows the impact of suicide firsthand. After losing colleagues to suicide, she dedicated herself to fighting this leading cause of death. Since earning her medical degree and training in psychiatry at the University of California, San Diego, Dr. Moutier has been a practicing psychiatrist, professor of psychiatry, dean in the medical school, medical director of the Inpatient Psychiatric Unit at the Veterans Affairs Medical Center in La Jolla, and has been clinically active with diverse patient populations, such as veterans, Asian refugee populations, as well as physicians and academic leaders with mental health conditions. She has presented at the White House, testified before the U.S. Congress on suicide prevention, and has appeared as an expert on *Anderson Cooper 360*, the BBC, *CBS This Morning*, *The Atlantic*, *The New York Times*, *Time*, *The Washington Post*, *The Economist*, and *NBC Nightly News*, among others.

Laurelle Myhra, Ph.D., LMFT, is Ojibwe and a enrolled member of Red Lake Nation and is the director of Behavioral Health at the Native American Community Clinic (NACC) and sits on the Health Equity Advisory & Leadership (HEAL) Council for the state of Minnesota and previously on the community board for Hennepin County Healthcare for the Homeless Clinic. Dr. Myhra completed her doctorate at the University of Minnesota in Family Social Science and Marriage and Family Therapy program, where she was an American Association for Marriage and Family Therapy Substance Abuse and Mental Health Services Administration Fellow. She has dedicated her career, as a researcher, supervisor, clinician, and educator, to addressing historical trauma, traumatic stress, and substance use disorders among Native Americans. She has published numerous peer-reviewed articles on these subjects. She has received training on the top evidence-based trauma treatment modalities, including Eye Movement Desensitization Reprocessing (EMDR), Trauma Focused Cognitive Behavioral Therapy (TF-CBT), and Honoring Children, Mending the Circle (culturally adapted TF-CBT) and has adapted these to be culturally appropriate in practice. She was also trained on White Bison's Wellbriety-Medicine Wheel and 12-Step, culturally adapted model, and Mending Broken Hearts on healing from grief and loss. Dr. Myhra is a licensed marriage and family therapist and has provided therapeutic service to the Native American community in the Twin Cities metro area since 2005.

Alfreda Patterson has worked in the counseling field since 1997 in positions ranging from Counselor Tech, Case Manager, and Substance Abuse Counselor. She was educated at Baltimore City Community College with a degree in Allied Human Services in Addiction Counseling. She joined Concerted Care Group on September 14, 2015. Her work as a substance use counselor and a housing coordinator is very dear to her heart. Her childhood and most of her adult life was in East Baltimore. She come from a background of Human Services: her mother was a teacher for 45 years, and her brother is a professor at Morgan State University. She owned several transitional houses for more than 7 years that housed clients with substance use disorders and mental health. Her goal is to always help anyone in need with services and adequate care. Housing is an important part of stabilization. When she is not working, she is working. She has been married for 27 years and is raising an 8-year-old with autism. Her message is always dedication, honesty, and commitment.

Joshua Prasad, M.P.H., is currently the director of the Concerted Care Group (CCG) integrated behavioral health and wellness center focused on addiction in Frederick, Maryland. At CCG, he is designing and implementing new programs to expand access to primary care and mental health in addition to traditional addiction and medication-assisted treatment. He is also currently a board member, and has been nominated as next-chair for a tobacco control and prevention nonprofit—Counter Tools. Mr. Prasad is also the co-founder of a social justice innovation consulting firm, IIF Health and is currently advising several disruptive companies domestically and internationally. He was formerly a senior advisor in the Office of the Assistant Secretary for Health within the Department of Health and Human Services (HHS) in Washington, DC. There he focused on increasing the incorporation of the social determinants of health through national initiatives, the development of health systems and workforce concerns for rural communities, and designed solutions to improve government efficiencies. While at HHS, he also assumed the role as director for the National Tobacco-Free College Campus Initiative, which designed policy and community-based solutions and provide technical assistance to increase tobacco-free environments. Prior to this time in the federal government, Mr. Prasad worked as an advocacy outreach worker at a community health center in Philadelphia, and performs epidemiological analyses at the State Department of Health in Pennsylvania. In 2015, he completed an Innovation Fellowship at the Harvard Medical School Center for Primary Care where he co-founded a startup focused on improving preventive health. Prior to this, he received his Master's in Public Health from Drexel University, and his bachelor's degree from Rutgers University, where he double majored in English and Psychology.

Jerry Reed, Ph.D., M.S.W., serves as the senior vice president for Practice Leadership at Education Development Center. In this capacity, he directs the Suicide, Violence and Injury Prevention Portfolio leading a staff of 53. He oversees the work on multiple projects such as the Suicide Prevention Resource Center, the Zero Suicide Institute, the Action Alliance for Suicide Prevention, the Children's Safety Network, several violence prevention initiatives and serves as co-director of the Injury Control Research Center for Suicide Prevention with partners at the University of Rochester Medical Center. His interests include geriatrics, mental health, suicide prevention, global violence prevention, and public policy. Dr. Reed recently co-led the committee that updated the U.S. National Strategy for Suicide Prevention and he serves as an Executive Committee member of the National Action Alliance for Suicide Prevention. Dr. Reed received a Ph.D. in Health Related Sciences with an emphasis in Gerontology from the Virginia Commonwealth University in Richmond in 2007 and his M.S.W. degree from University of Maryland at Baltimore in 1982 with an emphasis in Aging Administration. He served in the U.S. Navy during the period 1974–1978.

Jennifer Shaw, Ph.D., is a medical anthropologist and a senior researcher at Southcentral Foundation (SCF), an Alaska Native-owned and operated health care system serving 65,000 people in the greater Anchorage area and 55 rural villages. At SCF, Dr. Shaw's research has focused heavily on suicide prevention in the Alaska Native community, including Methamphetamine and Suicide Prevention Initiative projects to identify protective factors for suicide, explore lived experience of recovery from suicidal thoughts and behavior, and identify factors in the electronic health record associated with suicide risk. She is currently funded as the primary investigator on an Idea Networks of Biomedical Research Excellence–funded study to apply a predictive algorithm to electronic health records to stratify suicide risk. She is also the Alaska primary investigator of a National Institute of Mental

Health–funded four-site trial to culturally tailor and test Caring Contacts for suicide prevention.

Holly C. Wilcox, Ph.D., has a joint faculty appointment as an associate professor in the Johns Hopkins Bloomberg School of Public Health's Department of Mental Health and the Johns Hopkins University School of Medicine's Department of Psychiatry. Dr. Wilcox received her Ph.D. in Psychiatric Epidemiology from the Johns Hopkins Bloomberg School of Public Health. She just completed a national project to summarize the state of the science and research needs for data linkage, which served as the foundation for a National Institutes of Health Pathway to Prevention workshop on youth suicide prevention. She teaches a course in the Bloomberg School of Public Health titled "Suicide as a Public Health Problem" and leads a multidisciplinary, interdepartmental suicide prevention work group at Johns Hopkins.

T. J. Wocasek's first professional job was a substance use counselor at the Salvation Army Clitheroe Center (SACC) in Anchorage, Alaska, in 1998. In 2000, he was promoted to the Dual Diagnosis Supervisor at SACC where he served for 2.5 years. The clientele in this program had issues with mental illness, substance abuse, and homelessness. He has worked at Southcentral Foundation since 2002. Mr. Wocasek has worked as a clinician at the Southcentral Foundation Pathway Home for 4 years where he addressed behavioral health and substance abuse issues with adolescents in a residential treatment setting. He transferred to the Behavioral Urgent Response Team (BURT) as a clinician working with people who were in behavioral health crisis. He conducted risk assessments, assessed for depression and anxiety symptoms, completed substance use screenings, and consulted on capacity cases. In 2006, Mr. Wocasek started as a BURT clinician and was promoted to BURT clinical supervisor in 2007. He developed the BURT team into a 24/7 team. From 2006 to 2010, he had a private practice where he addressed behavioral health and substance abuse issues on an outpatient basis. From 2009 to 2010, Mr. Wocasek was the project director for two of Southcentral Foundation suicide prevention grants, the Substance Abuse and Mental Health Services Administration and the Indian Health Services Methamphetamine and Suicide Prevention Initiative. These grants are providing more resources for suicide prevention. From 2010 to 2015, he was the Pathway Home Clinical Supervisor. Since 2015, Mr. Wocasek has been the BURT Clinical Supervisor.

Keith Wood, Ph.D., ABPP, has a 40-year history of providing services to, creating and implementing programs for, and researching intervention effectiveness with individuals diagnosed with severe mental illness behavioral disorders. He developed and directed successful service programs in psychiatric inpatient and crisis stabilization units, psychiatric emergency rooms, hospital-affiliated outpatient behavioral health clinics, community mental health centers and on-the-street settings. Currently he is the clinical director of an intensive outpatient service focused on reducing psychotic symptoms through the teaching and enhancement of normalization and positive life functioning skills.

NATIONAL ACADEMIES STAFF AND CONSULTANTS

Natacha Blain, J.D., Ph.D., serves as the director of the Board on Children, Youth, and Families at the National Academies. Dr. Blain has more than 15 years of experience working with policy makers and senior legislative officials on a variety of social justice issues and campaigns, including serving as a Supreme Court Fellow, Chief Counsel to Senator Dick Durbin (D-IL) on the Senate Judiciary Committee, and Lead Strategic Advisor for the Children's Defense Fund's Cradle to Prison Pipeline Campaign. Most recently, she served as associate director/acting executive director at Grantmakers for Children, Youth and Families (GCYF). Dr. Blain joined GCYF in January 2010 as GCYF's first director of public policy. Her talents were quickly recognized and 1 year later, she was elevated to associate director. For approximately 2 years at the end of her tenure with GCYF, she also served as the acting executive director. In her various capacities, Dr. Blain has played a critical role in helping convene and engage diverse constituencies, fostering leadership, collaboration, and innovation-sharing through a network of funders committed to the enduring well-being of children, youth, and families.

Joseph Goodman is a senior program assistant and has been at the National Academies for 11 years. He has worked on a variety of activities related to military and veterans, Social Security, traumatic brain injury, and more.

Bridget B. Kelly, M.D., Ph.D., is a consultant specializing in strategy development, learning and evaluation, and meeting design and facilitation. She worked previously at the National Academies of Sciences, Engineering, and Medicine for 8 years leading a portfolio of projects that included mental health, early childhood, chronic diseases, HIV, and evaluation science, culminating in a term as the interim director of the Board on Children, Youth, and Families. More recently she co-founded the nonprofit Bridging Health & Community, with the mission of helping the health sector work more effectively with communities. She is also an experienced dancer, choreographer, and arts administrator. She received an M.D. and a Ph.D. from Duke University and a B.A. from Williams College.

Natalie Perou Lubin is a senior program assistant with the Board on Health Care Services and the National Cancer Policy Forum (NCPF) of the National Academies of Sciences, Engineering, and Medicine. Ms. Lubin has helped plan and disseminate NCPF workshops, including Long-Term Survivorship Care after Cancer Treatment, Establishing Effective Patient Navigation Programs in Oncology, and more. Prior to the National Academies, Ms. Lubin worked as a Program Assistant at the Duke-Margolis Center for Health Policy. In collaboration with the Duke-Margolis Center and the Duke Global Health Institute, she helped edit a policy report evaluating the funding mechanisms in global development. In Ms. Lubin's academic and professional career, she is passionate in the areas of child and maternal health, women empowerment, and education and its intersection with health. Supporting these interests, in the summer of 2016, Ms. Lubin was a data analyst intern at the Global Development Lab at the U.S. Agency for International Development, in which she worked on the monitoring, evaluation and learning strategy for the Innovations and Design Advisory team. Additionally, in the summer of 2015, Ms. Lubin carried out water sanitation research in rural Kenya through DukeEngage and the Women's Institute for Secondary Education and Research. Ms. Lubin is a graduate of Duke University with bachelor's degrees in Global Health and Cultural Anthropology.

Marc Meisnere, M.S.P.H., is an associate program officer at the National Academies of Sciences, Engineering, and Medicine's Board on Health Care Services. He currently works on activities related to clinician well-being, mental health, and primary care. Since 2010, Mr. Meisnere has worked on a variety National Academies' consensus studies, primarily focusing on mental health among service members and veterans. Before joining the National Academies, Mr. Meisnere worked on a family planning media project in northern Nigeria with the Johns Hopkins Center for Communication Programs and on a variety of international health policy issues at the Population Reference Bureau. He is a graduate of Colorado College and the Johns Hopkins Bloomberg School of Public Health.

Sharyl Nass, Ph.D., serves as the director of the Board on Health Care Services and the director of the National Cancer Policy Forum (NCPF) at the National Academies of Sciences, Engineering, and Medicine. The National Academies provide independent, objective analysis and advice to the nation to solve complex problems and inform public policy decisions related to science, technology, and medicine. To enable the best possible care for all patients, the Board undertakes scholarly analysis of the organization, financing, effectiveness, workforce, and delivery of health care, with emphasis on quality, cost, and accessibility. NCPF examines policy issues pertaining to the entire continuum of cancer research and care. For nearly two decades, Dr. Nass has worked on a broad range of health and science policy topics that includes the quality and safety of health care and clinical trials, developing technologies for precision medicine, and strategies for large-scale biomedical science. She has a Ph.D. in cell biology from Georgetown University and undertook postdoctoral training at the Johns Hopkins University School of Medicine, as well as a research fellowship at the Max Planck Institute in Germany. She also holds a B.S. and an M.S. from the University of Wisconsin–Madison. She has been the recipient of the Cecil Medal for Excellence in Health Policy Research, a Distinguished Service Award from the National Academies, and the Institute of Medicine staff team achievement award (as team leader).

Anne N. Styka, M.P.H., is a program officer in the Health and Medicine Division at the National Academies. Over her tenure she has worked on more than 10 studies on a broad range of topics related to the health of military and veteran populations. Studies have included mental health treatment offered in the Department of Defense and the Department of Veterans Affairs (VA), designing and evaluating epidemiological research studies using VA data for health outcomes related to deployment-related exposures including burn pits and chemicals, and directing a research program of fostering new research studies using data and biospecimens collected as part of the 20-year Air Force Health Study. Before coming to the National Academies, Ms. Styka spent several years working as an epidemiologist for the New Mexico Department of Health and the Albuquerque Area Southwest Tribal Epidemiology Center, and she spent several months in Zambia as the epidemiologist on a study of silicosis and other nonmalignant respiratory diseases among copper miners. She has several peer-reviewed publications and has contributed to numerous state and national reports. She received her B.S. in Cell and Tissue Bioengineering from the University of Illinois at Chicago and has an M.P.H. in Epidemiology from the University of Michigan. Ms. Styka was the 2017 recipient of the Division of Earth and Life Sciences Mt. Everest Award, the 2015 recipient of the Institute of Medicine and National Academy of Medicine Multitasker Award, and a member of the 2011 National Academies' Distinguished Group Award.